THE ULTIMA1
TYPE 2 DIABETES
COOKBOOK FOR
BEGINNERS

Cook Your Way to Better Health with 2000 Days of Flavorful, Low-Carb, and Low-Sugar Recipes, Complete with a Meal Plan for Diabetes Management

Camila Gray

Table of Contents

INTRODUCTION	**6**
TYPE 2 DIABETES	6
RISK FACTORS	8
IMPORTANCE OF MANAGEMENT	9
CHAPTER 1: LIST OF PERMITTED AND PROHIBITED FOODS	**11**
CHAPTER 2: BREAKFAST RECIPES	**13**
1. SMOKED SALMON AND CUCUMBER WRAP	13
2. ALMOND FLOUR PANCAKES	13
3. EGG AND VEGGIE BREAKFAST BURRITO	14
4. BANANA WALNUT MUFFINS	15
5. BERRY AND SPINACH SMOOTHIE BOWL	15
6. ZUCCHINI AND CHEESE EGG BAKE	16
7. OAT BRAN PORRIDGE WITH CINNAMON	17
8. VEGGIE OMELET MUFFINS	17
9. COTTAGE CHEESE PANCAKES	18
10. SPINACH AND MUSHROOM FRITTATA	18
11. OVERNIGHT OATS WITH NUTS AND BERRIES	19
12. TURKEY AND VEGGIE BREAKFAST SKILLET	20
13. APPLE CINNAMON QUINOA PORRIDGE	20
14. QUINOA BREAKFAST BOWL	21
15. AVOCADO AND EGG TOAST	21
16. TOMATO BASIL MOZZARELLA FRITTATA	22
17. WHOLE GRAIN TOAST WITH AVOCADO AND TOMATO	23
18. CAULIFLOWER HASH BROWNS	23
19. PEANUT BUTTER BANANA SMOOTHIE	24
20. MEXICAN BREAKFAST CASSEROLE	24
CHAPTER 3: LUNCH RECIPES	**26**
1. GRILLED CHICKEN SALAD WITH VINAIGRETTE	26
2. TURKEY LETTUCE WRAPS	27
3. QUINOA AND BLACK BEAN STUFFED PEPPERS	27
4. MEDITERRANEAN CHICKPEA SALAD	28
5. SALMON AND ASPARAGUS FOIL PACKETS	29
6. SPINACH AND FETA TURKEY BURGER	29
7. CAULIFLOWER RICE STIR-FRY WITH TOFU	30
8. TURKEY AND AVOCADO WRAP	31
9. SHRIMP AND VEGETABLE SKEWERS	31
10. TOMATO BASIL CHICKEN WRAP	32
11. BROCCOLI AND CHICKEN QUICHE	33
12. CUCUMBER AND RADISH SALAD WITH FETA	33
13. MINESTRONE SOUP WITH WHOLE WHEAT PASTA	34

14. Grilled Veggie and Hummus Wrap 35

15. Pesto Zoodles with Cherry Tomatoes 36

16. Tuna Salad Lettuce Wraps 36

17. Chicken and Vegetable Kabobs 37

18. Caprese Salad with Balsamic Glaze 38

19. Eggplant and Chickpea Stew 38

20. Turkey and Spinach Stuffed Mushrooms 39

CHAPTER 4: Dinner Recipes **40**

1. Baked Lemon Herb Chicken 40

2. Quinoa-Stuffed Bell Peppers 40

3. Garlic Parmesan Baked Cod 41

4. Cauliflower and Lentil Curry 42

5. Greek Quinoa Salad 42

6. Grilled Salmon with Dill Sauce 43

7. Zucchini Noodles with Pesto and Cherry Tomatoes 44

8. Lemon Garlic Shrimp Skewers 45

9. Chicken and Broccoli Casserole 45

10. Spinach and Feta Stuffed Chicken Breast 46

11. Chickpea and Vegetable Curry 47

12. Teriyaki Tofu Stir-Fry 47

13. Mediterranean Baked Fish 48

14. Spaghetti Squash with Tomato Basil Sauce 49

15. Pesto Chicken with Roasted Vegetables 50

16. Baked Zucchini Boats with Ground Turkey 50

17. Lentil and Spinach Soup 51

18. Grilled Vegetable and Quinoa Bowl 52

19. Turkey and Vegetable Skillet 53

20. Broiled Lemon Garlic Tilapia 53

CHAPTER 5: Snack Recipes **55**

1. Veggie Sticks with Hummus 55

2. Almonds and Walnuts Mix 55

3. Hard-Boiled Eggs with Cherry Tomatoes 56

4. Apple Slices with Peanut Butter 56

5. Roasted Chickpeas with Spices 56

6. Edamame with Sea Salt 57

7. Avocado Salsa with Whole Wheat Crackers 57

8. Trail Mix with Nuts and Seeds 58

9. Cherry Almond Energy Bites 58

10. Cucumber and Tomato Salad 59

11. Mini Caprese Skewers 60

12. Baked Kale Chips 60

13. Sliced Bell Peppers with Guacamole 61

14. Greek Salad Skewers 61

15. Quinoa and Black Bean Salad Cups 62

16. Smoked Salmon Cucumber Bites 62

17. Celery Sticks with Cream Cheese 63

18. Roasted Pumpkin Seeds 63

19. Whole Grain Rice Cake with Cottage Cheese 64

20. Eggplant Lasagna 64

CHAPTER 6: Dessert Recipes **66**

1. Baked Apples with Cinnamon 66

2. Dark Chocolate-Dipped Strawberries 66

3. Coconut Flour Banana Bread 67

4. Almond Flour Blueberry Muffins 67

5. Chocolate Avocado Mousse 68

6. Pumpkin Spice Chia Seed Pudding 69

7. Mixed Berry Sorbet 69

8. Vanilla Bean Panna Cotta 70

9. Lemon Poppy Seed Almond Cake 70

10. Ricotta and Berry Parfait 71

11. Pistachio and Cranberry Biscotti 71

12. Greek Yogurt and Honey Frozen Drops 72

13. Avocado Lime Cheesecake Bites 73

14. Almond and Coconut Energy Balls 73

15. Baked Pears with Cinnamon and Walnuts 74

16. Raspberry Almond Crumble Bars 74

17. Cinnamon Roasted Almonds 75

18. Coconut and Lime Sorbet 76

19. Strawberry and Mint Infused Water 76

20. Pecan and Date Energy Squares 77

Shopping List **78**

30 Day Meal Plan **80**

Conversion Table **82**

Conclusion **85**

Introduction

In the United States, diabetes stands as the seventh most prevalent cause of death, impacting around 30.3 million Americans, roughly constituting 9.4% of the population. Approximately one-third of Americans experience prediabetes, with 90% being unaware of their condition. In the absence of adequate nutrition, exercise, and weight control, 15-30% of individuals with prediabetes are at risk of developing type 2 diabetes within a five-year timeframe.

A diabetes diagnosis doesn't necessitate giving up favorite foods or making sacrifices for family members. Instead, adopting a healthy eating lifestyle is crucial to prevent health complications, especially if there's a family history of diabetes. If diagnosed with diabetes, there's no need to panic; by adhering to appropriate nutritional guidelines and working closely with a doctor, it's possible to lead a normal and healthy life.

The cornerstone of diabetes management lies in dietary choices. By effectively managing blood sugar levels through better food choices and portion control, the need for medication can be minimized or eliminated altogether. This book offers insights into diabetes, methods for prevention or management, and a collection of delicious and healthful recipes.

Type 2 Diabetes

This encompasses all types of diabetes arising from insufficient insulin secretion by the pancreatic beta cells in the islets of Langerhans, resistance of the body's tissues to insulin action (referred to as insulin resistance). It constitutes the predominant form of diabetes, making up approximately 90% of all cases of the disease. The cause is still unknown; although the pancreas is certainly capable of producing insulin, the body's cells cannot use it. The disease usually manifests itself after 30-40 years, and numerous risk factors associated with its onset have been recognized. These include a family history of diabetes, lack of physical exercise, being overweight, and belonging to certain ethnic groups. As for familiarity, about 40% of type 2 diabetics have first-degree relatives (parents, siblings) affected by the same disease, while in monozygotic twins, the concordance of the disease is close to 100%, suggesting a strong hereditary component for this type of diabetes. There are also rare forms of type 2 diabetes, known as MODY (Maturity Onset Diabetes of the Young), in which type 2 diabetes has a juvenile-onset, and rare genetic defects in the intracellular mechanisms of insulin action have been identified.

Type 2 diabetes is usually not diagnosed for many years, as hyperglycemia develops gradually and is not severe enough at first to give the classic symptoms of diabetes. Diagnosis usually occurs by chance or in conjunction with a situation of physical stress, such as infections or surgery. The likelihood of disease onset rises with advancing age, obesity, and insufficient physical activity. This observation suggests the potential for "primary" prevention strategies. These interventions aim to thwart the emergence of the disease and pivot on adopting a suitable lifestyle, encompassing nutritional considerations and regular physical exercise.

Causes of Type 2 Diabetes?

The number of cases of Type 2 diabetes is soaring, related to the obesity epidemic. Type 2 diabetes occurs over time and involves problems getting enough sugar (glucose) into the body's cells. Overweight or obese is the greatest risk factor for Type 2 diabetes. However, the risk is higher if the concentration of weight is around the abdomen as opposed to the thighs and hips. The belly fat that surrounds the liver and abdominal organs are closely linked to insulin resistance. Calories obtained from everyday sugary drinks such as energy drinks, soda, coffee drinks, and processed foods like muffins, doughnuts, cereal, and candy could greatly increase the weight around your abdomen. Apart from maintaining a healthy diet, reducing the consumption of sugary foods can lead to a trimmer waistline and a decreased likelihood of developing diabetes.

Symptoms of Type 2 Diabetes

Type 2 diabetes is a chronic condition that can develop gradually over time, and its symptoms may vary from person to person. Some individuals may experience mild or no symptoms initially, while others may have more pronounced signs. It's important to recognize the symptoms of type 2 diabetes because an early diagnosis can lead to effective management and prevention of complications. Here are some common symptoms associated with type 2 diabetes:

- **Increased Thirst and Frequent Urination:** Excessive thirst, known as polydipsia, is a common symptom of type 2 diabetes. The body tries to eliminate extra glucose through urine, leading to increased urine production and subsequently frequent urination (polyuria). Individuals may notice they need to urinate more frequently, especially at night (nocturia).
- **Fatigue and Weakness:** Type 2 diabetes can cause a persistent feeling of tiredness and lack of energy. The body's inability to effectively utilize glucose for energy can lead to fatigue and weakness. Individuals may feel exhausted even after getting adequate rest.
- **Unexplained Weight Loss or Gain:** Sudden weight loss can occur in some cases of type 2 diabetes, despite increased appetite. This happens when the body can't use glucose properly, so it starts breaking down fat and muscle tissue for energy. On the other hand, some individuals may experience weight gain due to insulin resistance & metabolic changes.
- **Increased Hunger:** Despite eating regularly, individuals with type 2 diabetes may experience persistent hunger (polyphagia). The body's cells may not be receiving enough glucose, leading to increased appetite and food cravings.
- **Blurred Vision:** High blood sugar levels can affect the lenses in the eyes, leading to changes in vision. Blurred vision is a common symptom of untreated or poorly managed diabetes. It may take longer for the eyes to adjust to changes in focus, causing difficulties with near or distant vision.
- **Slow Healing of Wounds:** High blood sugar levels can impair the body's ability to heal wounds and fight infections. Cuts, sores, or bruises may take longer to heal, and individuals with type 2 diabetes may be more prone to infections, particularly in the feet and skin.
- **Frequent Infections:** Type 2 diabetes can weaken the immune system, making individuals more susceptible to infections. Common infections include urinary tract infections (UTIs), yeast infections (particularly in women), and skin infections. These infections may occur more frequently or be more challenging to treat.
- **Tingling or Numbness:** Elevated blood sugar levels can damage the nerves, leading to a condition called diabetic neuropathy. Tingling, numbness, or a burning sensation may occur in the hands, feet, or legs. This symptom is often one of the first signs of nerve damage due to diabetes.
- **Dry Skin and Itching:** Diabetes can cause dry skin due to dehydration and poor circulation. The skin may become dry and itchy, particularly in the lower legs and feet. Itching can be persistent and bothersome, leading to scratching and potential skin infections.

- **Darkened Skin Patches:** Some individuals with type 2 diabetes may develop acanthosis nigricans, a condition characterized by darkened and thickened patches of skin, usually around the neck, armpits, or groin. This condition is associated with insulin resistance.

It's important to note that these symptoms can also be present in other health conditions, and some individuals with type 2 diabetes may not experience any symptoms at all. Therefore, it's crucial to consult a healthcare professional for an accurate diagnosis if you suspect you may have diabetes.

Risk Factors

Type 2 diabetes is a multifaceted condition shaped by a blend of genetic, environmental, and lifestyle factors. Recognizing the risk factors linked to the onset of type 2 diabetes is crucial for pinpointing individuals who might be at an elevated risk and implementing preventive measures. Here are some key risk factors that contribute to the development of type 2 diabetes:

- **Obesity:** One of the foremost risk factors for type 2 diabetes is obesity. The presence of extra body fat, especially visceral fat concentrated around the abdomen, is strongly linked to insulin resistance. Insulin resistance is a condition wherein cells become less responsive to the effects of insulin. Adipose tissue, or fat cells, release chemicals that can interfere with insulin's action, leading to impaired glucose regulation. The more extra weight an individual carries, the higher their risk of developing insulin resistance and type 2 diabetes.
- **Genetic Predisposition:** Genetics plays a role in the development of type 2 diabetes. Having a family history of the condition increases the likelihood of developing it. Certain genetic variants can affect how the body processes glucose and how insulin functions. However, genetics alone is not the sole determinant of type 2 diabetes. Lifestyle factors also wield considerable influence, and individuals with a family history of diabetes can mitigate their risk by embracing healthy lifestyle habits.
- **Lack of Physical Activity:** Physical inactivity is a significant risk factor for type 2 diabetes. Consistent physical activity enhances insulin sensitivity and encourages glucose uptake by the muscles, resulting in lower blood sugar levels. Conversely, a sedentary lifestyle can contribute to weight gain, insulin resistance, and an elevated risk of developing diabetes. Engaging in moderate-intensity aerobic activities, such as brisk walking, cycling, or swimming, for a minimum of 150 mins per week can markedly decrease the risk of type 2 diabetes.
- **Poor Diet:** Unhealthy eating habits, particularly a diet high in refined carbohydrates, added sugars, and saturated and trans fats, increase the risk of type 2 diabetes. These dietary factors contribute to weight gain, promote inflammation, and impair insulin sensitivity. Consuming a well-balanced diet that includes ample fruits, vegetables, lean proteins, whole grains, and healthy fats contributes to stabilizing blood sugar levels and lowers the likelihood of diabetes onset. Additionally, excessive consumption of sugary beverages, such as soda and fruit juices, is strongly associated with an increased risk of type 2 diabetes.
- **Age:** The likelihood of developing type 2 diabetes rises with advancing age. While this condition can manifest at any point in life, it predominantly impacts individuals aged 45 and above. The heightened susceptibility in older adults could stem from a blend of factors, encompassing diminished physical activity, elevated body weight, and alterations in hormone levels influencing glucose metabolism. However, it is important to note that type 2 diabetes is increasingly being diagnosed in younger individuals due to rising rates of obesity and sedentary lifestyles.
- **Gestational Diabetes:** Women who have had gestational diabetes during pregnancy face an elevated risk of developing type 2 diabetes in the future. Gestational diabetes is a temporary condition occurring when the body can't produce sufficient insulin to meet increased demands during pregnancy. The

occurrence of gestational diabetes signals an augmented likelihood of developing type 2 diabetes later on. Furthermore, offspring born to mothers with gestational diabetes carry a heightened risk of obesity and type 2 diabetes as they age.

- **Ethnicity:** Certain ethnic groups have a higher predisposition to type 2 diabetes. Individuals with African, Hispanic, Asian, and Indigenous backgrounds have a higher likelihood of experiencing this condition when compared to those of European descent. The underlying reasons for these disparities remain not fully comprehended, but it is probable that a mix of genetic, environmental, and lifestyle factors contributes. Furthermore, people from these ethnic groups may exhibit a greater susceptibility to obesity and insulin resistance, thereby amplifying their vulnerability to developing type 2 diabetes.

- **High Blood Pressure and Cardiovascular Disease:** Individuals with high blood pressure (hypertension) or a history of cardiovascular disease are at an increased risk of developing type 2 diabetes. Hypertension and cardiovascular disease share common risk factors with type 2 diabetes, such as obesity, physical inactivity, and poor diet. Furthermore, these conditions often coexist and can exacerbate each other's negative effects on overall health.

- **Polycystic Ovary Syndrome (PCOS):** Polycystic ovary syndrome (PCOS) is a hormonal imbalance affecting women in their reproductive years. Symptoms include irregular menstrual cycles, excessive hair growth, and the presence of cysts on the ovaries. PCOS is strongly linked to insulin resistance, elevating the likelihood of developing type 2 diabetes. Women with PCOS should be vigilant about managing their weight, adopting a healthy diet, and engaging in regular physical activity to lower their risk of developing diabetes.

- **Sleep Disorders:** Sleep disorders, such as obstructive sleep apnea and insomnia, have been linked to an increased risk of type 2 diabetes. Disrupted sleep patterns and inadequate sleep duration can impair insulin sensitivity and glucose metabolism, increasing the risk of developing diabetes. Addressing sleep disorders and ensuring adequate and restful sleep is an important aspect of diabetes prevention.

It's important to note that while these risk factors increase the likelihood of developing type 2 diabetes, they do not guarantee that an individual will develop the condition. Many people with one or more of these risk factors do not develop diabetes, while others without apparent risk factors may still develop the condition.

Importance of Management

Managing type 2 diabetes is crucial for maintaining overall health and preventing long-term complications. Here are key points emphasizing the importance of managing type 2 diabetes through a balanced diet, physical exercise, and prescribed medications:

1. **Blood Glucose Control:** Effective management helps control blood glucose levels, preventing them from reaching dangerous highs or lows. Consistent blood glucose control is essential for minimizing the risk of complications.

2. **Prevention of Complications:** Long-term complications of uncontrolled type 2 diabetes can be severe, including heart disease, kidney damage, nerve damage, and vision problems. Managing diabetes helps reduce the risk of these complications and improves overall quality of life.

3. **Balanced Diet:** A well-balanced diet is a cornerstone of diabetes management. Controlling carbohydrate intake, focusing on whole foods, and paying attention to portion sizes can help regulate blood sugar levels. A diet rich in fiber, lean proteins, fruits, vegetables, and whole grains supports overall health.

4. **Physical Exercise:** Regular physical activity is crucial for effectively managing type 2 diabetes. Engaging in exercise aids in reducing blood sugar levels, enhancing insulin sensitivity, and supporting weight management. It also contributes to cardiovascular health, reducing the risk of heart-related complications.

5. **Medication Adherence:** In some cases, prescribed medications, including oral medications or insulin, may be necessary to manage blood glucose levels effectively. Adhering to the prescribed medication regimen as directed by healthcare professionals is crucial for optimal diabetes control.

6. **Lifestyle Modifications:** Lifestyle modifications, such as quitting smoking and limiting alcohol intake, play a significant role in diabetes management. These changes contribute to better overall health and assist in controlling blood sugar levels.

7. **Regular Monitoring and Check-ups:** Routine monitoring of blood glucose levels and regular check-ups with healthcare providers are essential components of diabetes management. These measures help detect any deviations from the target range and allow for timely adjustments to the treatment plan.

8. **Improved Energy Levels and Well-Being:** Effective diabetes management often leads to improved energy levels, better mood, and an overall sense of well-being. Keeping your blood sugar steady helps you have consistent energy all day long.

9. **Empowerment and Self-Care:** Managing type 2 diabetes empowers individuals to take control of their health through self-care practices. Education about the condition and its management helps individuals make informed decisions about their lifestyle, diet, and treatment options.

10. **Long-Term Health and Longevity:** By prioritizing diabetes management, individuals can significantly enhance their long-term health and increase their chances of leading a longer, healthier life.

CHAPTER 1: List of Permitted and Prohibited Foods

A well-balanced diet is crucial for managing type 2 diabetes effectively. Making informed food choices can help regulate blood glucose levels, promote weight management, and reduce the risk of complications. Here's a comprehensive guide to foods to include and avoid in a type 2 diabetes diet:

Foods to Eat:

1. **Whole Grains:** Opt for whole grains like brown rice, quinoa, oats, and whole wheat bread. These choices provide fiber, which helps regulate blood sugar levels and promotes satiety.

2. **Vegetables:** Diversify your vegetable intake with colorful options like leafy greens, broccoli, cauliflower, peppers, and tomatoes. These non-starchy vegetables are rich in vitamins, minerals, and fiber.

3. **Lean Proteins:** Choose lean protein sources to support muscle health and maintain steady energy levels. Examples include skinless poultry, fish, tofu, legumes, and low-fat dairy products.

4. **Fruits:** While fruits contain natural sugars, they also provide essential nutrients and fiber. Opt for whole fruits like berries, apples, and citrus fruits. Be mindful of portion sizes to manage carbohydrate intake.

5. **Healthy Fats:** Include healthy fats from avocados, nuts, seeds, and olive oil. They can improve insulin sensitivity and support heart health.

6. **Fatty Fish:** Eat fatty fish like salmon, mackerel, and trout for omega-3 fatty acids that fight inflammation and lower heart disease risk.

7. **Legumes:** Boost your fiber and protein intake with legumes like beans, lentils, and chickpeas, known for their low glycemic index that helps stabilize blood sugar levels.

8. **Dairy or Dairy Alternatives:** Choose low-fat or fat-free dairy products or fortified dairy alternatives like almond or soy milk. These provide essential nutrients like calcium and vitamin D without excessive saturated fats.

9. **Herbs and Spices:** Use herbs and spices like cinnamon, turmeric, and garlic to include flavor. Some may even help control blood sugar.

10. **Water:** Stay well-hydrated with water. Limit sugary beverages, as they can lead to spikes in blood sugar levels.

Foods to Limit or Avoid:

1. **Sugary Foods and Beverages:** Minimize the consumption of sugary foods and drinks, including candies, sodas, fruit juices, and desserts. These can cause rapid spikes in blood glucose levels.

2. **Processed Carbohydrates:** Reduce intake of refined carbohydrates like white bread, pasta, and sugary cereals. Choose whole grains for better blood sugar control.

3. **Saturated and Trans Fats:** Don't eat too much of the fats in fried foods, snacks, and certain baked goods. These fats can make it harder for your body to use insulin and can cause heart problems.

4. **High-Sodium Foods:** Watch your sodium intake, as it can affect blood pressure. Limit processed and salty foods, and opt for herbs and spices to flavor meals instead.

5. **Red and Processed Meats:** Don't eat too much red or processed meats, as they might increase your chances of getting diabetes and heart problems. Choose leaner proteins more often.

6. **Alcohol:** Consume alcohol in moderation, if at all. Excessive alcohol intake can affect blood sugar levels and interfere with medication.

7. **Full-Fat Dairy:** While dairy is beneficial, choose low-fat or fat-free options to reduce saturated fat intake.

8. **Portion Control:** Be mindful of portion sizes to avoid overeating, which can lead to spikes in blood sugar levels. Use smaller plates and pay attention to hunger and fullness cues.

9. **Hidden Sugars:** Check food labels for hidden sugars, as they can be present in unexpected places like condiments, sauces, and even some seemingly healthy snacks.

10. **White Potatoes and Refined Grains:** Limit the consumption of white potatoes and refined grains, as they can cause rapid spikes in blood sugar. Choose alternatives like sweet potatoes and whole grains.

CHAPTER 2: Breakfast Recipes

1.   Smoked Salmon and Cucumber Wrap

Preparation time: 10 mins

Cooking time: 0 mins

Servings: 2

Ingredients:

- 4 whole grain or low-carb tortillas
- 8 oz. smoked salmon (227 g)
- 1 cucumber, finely sliced
- 1/2 cup Greek yogurt (120 ml)
- 1 tbsp fresh dill, chopped (15 ml)
- 1 tsp lemon juice (5 ml)
- Salt and pepper as required

Directions:

1. Inside your container, mix Greek yogurt, salt, fresh dill, lemon juice, and pepper to create the sauce.
2. Lay out tortillas and spread a generous layer of the sauce on each.
3. Evenly distribute smoked salmon and cucumber slices on each tortilla.
4. Roll up the tortillas into wraps.
5. Cut in half diagonally and present.

Per serving: 300 kcal; Fat: 10g; Carbs: 25g; Protein: 25g; Fiber: 4g; Sugar: 3g; Sodium: 700mg; Glycemic Index: 30

---

2.   Almond Flour Pancakes

Preparation time: 10 mins

Cooking time: 10 mins

Servings: 2

Ingredients:

- 1 cup almond flour (96 g)
- 2 eggs
- 1/2 cup unsweetened almond milk (120 ml)
- 1 tbsp coconut oil, melted (15 ml)
- 1 tsp baking powder (5 ml)
- 1/2 tsp vanilla extract (2.5 ml)

Directions:

1. Inside your container, whisk together almond flour, eggs, almond milk, dissolved coconut oil, baking powder, and vanilla extract till smooth.
2. Warm a non-stick griddle in a middling temp.
3. Pour 1/4 cup of batter into your griddle for every pancake.
4. Cook the food till bubbles appear on the surface, then turn it over and continue cooking it till the remaining half is golden brown.
5. Perform the same steps using the remainder batter.
6. Present with a sprinkle of your sugar-free maple syrup or fresh berries.

Per serving: 320 kcal; Fat: 26g; Carbs: 10g; Protein: 14g; Fiber: 4g; Sugar: 2g; Sodium: 320mg; Glycemic Index: 20

3.   Egg and Veggie Breakfast Burrito

Preparation time: 15 mins

Cooking time: 10 mins

Servings: 2

Ingredients:

- 4 whole grain or low-carb tortillas
- 4 big eggs, scrambled
- 1 cup mixed veggies (bell peppers, onions, spinach) (about 150 g)
- 1/2 cup black beans, drained and washed (120 g)
- 1/2 cup salsa (sugar-free) (120 ml)
- 1/4 cup torn low-fat cheese (30 g)
- Salt and pepper as required
- Cooking spray for greasing

Directions:

1. Inside your griddle, sauté mixed veggies till softened.
2. Include scrambled eggs to the griddle then cook 'til done.
3. Warm tortillas in a separate pan or microwave.
4. Assemble the burritos by layering eggs and veggies, black beans, salsa, and torn cheese onto each tortilla.
5. Fold the sides then roll up the tortillas into burritos.
6. Optional: mildly grill the burritos on each side for a crispier texture.
7. Present warm.

Per serving: 380 kcal; Fat: 14g; Carbs: 40g; Protein: 20g; Fiber: 10g; Sugar: 4g; Sodium: 600mg; Glycemic Index: 25

4.   Banana Walnut Muffins

Preparation time: 15 mins

Cooking time: 20 mins

Servings: 12

Ingredients:

- 2 cups almond flour (192 g)
- 1 tsp baking powder (5 ml)
- 1/2 tsp baking soda (2.5 ml)
- 1/4 tsp salt (1.25 ml)
- 1 tsp ground cinnamon (5 ml)
- 3 ripe bananas, mashed (about 360 g)
- 3 big eggs
- 1/4 cup coconut oil, melted (60 ml)
- 1 tsp vanilla extract (5 ml)
- 1/2 cup chopped walnuts (60 g)

Directions:

1. Warm up the oven to 350 deg.F.(180 deg.C.) then line your muffin tin with paper liners.
2. Inside your container, whisk together almond flour, baking powder, baking soda, salt, and cinnamon.
3. Inside a distinct container, mix mashed bananas, eggs, dissolved coconut oil, and vanilla extract.
4. Blend wet & dry components, mixing till blended.
5. Fold in chopped walnuts.
6. Spoon batter into your muffin cups, around two-thirds of all of them being filled.
7. Bake for 20 mins or till someone inserts a toothpick and it comes out spotless.
8. Leave the muffins to settle prior to presenting.

Per serving: 220 kcal; Fat: 18g; Carbs: 10g; Protein: 7g; Fiber: 3g; Sugar: 4g; Sodium: 180mg; Glycemic Index: 35

---

5.   Berry and Spinach Smoothie Bowl

Preparation time: 10 mins

Cooking time: 0 mins

Servings: 2

Ingredients:

- 2 cups fresh spinach leaves (60 g)
- 1 cup mixed berries (e.g., strawberries, blueberries, raspberries) (150 g)
- 1 ripe banana
- 1/2 cup unsweetened almond milk (120 ml)

- 1 tbsp chia seeds (12 g)

Toppings:
- Sliced almonds
- Torn coconut
- Fresh berries

Directions:
1. Inside a mixer, blend spinach, mixed berries, banana, and almond milk.
2. Blend till smooth.
3. Pour the smoothie into containers.
4. Top with chia seeds, sliced almonds, torn coconut, and fresh berries.
5. Present instantly and relish with a spoon.

Per serving: 180 kcal; Fat: 7g; Carbs: 26g; Protein: 5g; Fiber: 8g; Sugar: 12g; Sodium: 80mg; Glycemic Index: 30

---

6.   Zucchini and Cheese Egg Bake

Preparation time: 15 mins

Cooking time: 25 mins

Servings: 4

Ingredients:
- 2 medium zucchinis, grated (about 300 g)
- 1 cup torn low-fat cheese (120 g)
- 6 big eggs
- 1/4 cup almond flour (30 g)
- 1/4 cup unsweetened almond milk (60 ml)
- 1 tsp olive oil (5 ml)
- 1/2 tsp baking powder (2.5 ml)
- Salt and pepper as required
- Fresh herbs for garnish (optional)

Directions:
1. Warm up the oven to 375 deg.F.(190 deg.C.) then oil your baking dish with olive oil.
2. Inside your container, blend grated zucchini, torn cheese, eggs, almond flour, almond milk, baking powder, salt, and pepper.
3. Pour solution into your prepared baking dish.
4. Bake for 25 mins or 'til the top is golden and the eggs are set.
5. Allow it to rest mildly, then slice then garnish with fresh herbs if anticipated.

Per serving: 220 kcal; Fat: 15g; Carbs: 8g; Protein: 14g; Fiber: 2g; Sugar: 4g; Sodium: 280mg; Glycemic Index: 20

7.   Oat Bran Porridge with Cinnamon

Preparation time: 5 mins

Cooking time: 10 mins

Servings: 2

Ingredients:

- 1 cup oat bran (94 g)
- 2 cups water (480 ml)
- 1/2 tsp ground cinnamon (2.5 ml)
- 1 tbsp flax seeds (7 g)
- 1/4 cup unsweetened almond milk (60 ml)
- Fresh berries for topping (optional)

Directions:

1. Inside your saucepot, heat the water until it boils.
2. Stir in oat bran, decrease temp. to low, then simmer for 5-7 mins, mixing irregularly.
3. Include ground cinnamon and flaxseeds, mixing till well blended.
4. Take out from temp. and allow it to relax for a couple of mins.
5. Split the porridge into containers, sprinkle with almond milk, and top using fresh berries if anticipated.
6. Present warm.

Per serving: 180 kcal; Fat: 5g; Carbs: 32g; Protein: 8g; Fiber: 8g; Sugar: 2g; Sodium: 10mg; Glycemic Index: 45

---

8.   Veggie Omelet Muffins

Preparation time: 10 mins

Cooking time: 20 mins

Servings: 4

Ingredients:

- 6 eggs
- 1/2 cup cubed bell peppers (75 g)
- 1/2 cup cubed tomatoes (75 g)
- 1/4 cup cubed onions (40 g)
- 1/4 cup chopped spinach (30 g)
- Salt and pepper as required
- Cooking spray

Directions:

1. Warm up the oven to 350 deg.F.(180 deg.C.) then oil your muffin tin with cooking sprinkle.
2. Inside your container, whisk the eggs then flavour using salt and pepper.

3. Stir in bell peppers, tomatoes, onions, and chopped spinach.
4. Pour the egg solution uniformlyinto your muffin cups.
5. Bake for 20 mins or 'til the muffins are set and mildly golden.
6. Allow them to cool for a couple of mins prior to presenting.

Per serving: 150 kcal; Fat: 10g; Carbs: 4g; Protein: 12g; Fiber: 1g; Sugar: 2g; Sodium: 120mg; Glycemic Index: 20

---

9. Cottage Cheese Pancakes

Preparation time: 10 mins

Cooking time: 10 mins

Servings: 3

Ingredients:

- 1 cup low-fat cottage cheese (240 g)
- 2 eggs
- 1/2 cup whole wheat flour (60 g)
- 1 tsp baking powder (5 ml)
- 1 tsp vanilla extract (5 ml)
- Cooking spray for greasing

Directions:

1. Inside a mixer, blend cottage cheese, eggs, whole wheat flour, baking powder, and vanilla extract. Blend till smooth.
2. Warm a non-stick griddle in a middling temp. and mildly coat with cooking sprinkle.
3. Pour 1/4 cup of batter into your griddle for every pancake.
4. Cook the food till bubbles appear on the surface, then turn it over and continue cooking it till the remaining half is golden brown.
5. Perform the same steps using the remainder batter.
6. Present with your fresh berries or a dollop of Greek yogurt if anticipated.

Per serving: 220 kcal; Fat: 6g; Carbs: 22g; Protein: 18g; Fiber: 3g; Sugar: 4g; Sodium: 380mg; Glycemic Index: 35

---

10. Spinach and Mushroom Frittata

Preparation time: 10 mins

Cooking time: 15 mins

Servings: 3

Ingredients:

- 6 eggs
- 1 cup fresh spinach, chopped (30 g)
- 1/2 cup mushrooms, sliced (75 g)
- 1/4 cup cubed onions (40 g)
- 1 piece garlic, crushed
- 1 tbsp olive oil (15 ml)
- Salt and pepper as required

Directions:

1. Warm up the oven to 350 deg.F.(180 deg.C.)
2. Inside your griddle, sauté mushrooms, onions, and garlic in olive oil till softened.
3. Include chopped spinach then cook 'til wilted.
4. Inside your container, beat the eggs then flavour using salt and pepper.
5. Pour egg solution over the vegetables in your griddle.
6. Cook on your stovetop for 2-3 mins, then transfer to the warmed up oven.
7. Bake for 12-15 mins or 'til the frittata is set and mildly golden.
8. Slice and present.

Per serving: 180 kcal; Fat: 12g; Carbs: 5g; Protein: 14g; Fiber: 2g; Sugar: 2g; Sodium: 180mg; Glycemic Index: 25

---

11. Overnight Oats with Nuts and Berries

Preparation time: 5 mins

Cooking time: 0 mins

Servings: 2

Ingredients:

- 1 cup old-fashioned oats (90 g)
- 1 cup unsweetened almond milk (240 ml)
- 1/2 cup mixed berries (e.g., blueberries, raspberries) (75 g)
- 2 tbsps chopped nuts (e.g., almonds, walnuts) (30 g)
- 1 tbsp chia seeds (12 g)
- 1 tsp honey (optional for sweetness) (5 ml)
- A dash of cinnamon

Directions:

1. Inside a jar or container, blend oats, almond milk, berries, chopped nuts, chia seeds, and honey (if using).
2. Blend thoroughly, ensuring oats are fully immersed in almond milk.
3. Put in the fridge overnight.
4. In the morning, give it a good stir, sprinkle with cinnamon, and relish the cold.

Per serving: 280 kcal; Fat: 12g; Carbs: 36g; Protein: 9g; Fiber: 8g; Sugar: 6g; Sodium: 80mg; Glycemic Index: 40

---

12. Turkey and Veggie Breakfast Skillet

Preparation time: 10 mins

Cooking time: 15 mins

Servings: 2

Ingredients:

- 1/2 lb. lean ground turkey (227 g)
- 1 bell pepper, cubed (about 150 g)
- 1 zucchini, cubed (about 200 g)
- 1 cup cherry tomatoes, halved (150 g)
- 1 tsp olive oil (5 ml)
- 1 tsp smoked paprika (5 ml)
- Salt and pepper as required
- 4 eggs
- Fresh parsley for garnish

Directions:

1. Warm olive oil in your griddle in a middling temp.
2. Include ground turkey then cook 'til browned.
3. Include bell pepper, zucchini, and cherry tomatoes to the griddle. Cook 'til vegetables are soft.
4. Flavour with smoked paprika, salt, and pepper.
5. Create wells in the solution and crack eggs into each well.
6. Cover the griddle then cook 'til eggs are done to your liking.
7. Decorate with fresh parsley as a finishing touch and present hot.

Per serving: 320 kcal; Fat: 18g; Carbs: 14g; Protein: 27g; Fiber: 4g; Sugar: 8g; Sodium: 340mg; Glycemic Index: 30

---

13. Apple Cinnamon Quinoa Porridge

Preparation time: 10 mins

Cooking time: 15 mins

Servings: 2

Ingredients:

- 1/2 cup quinoa, washed (85 g)
- 1 cup unsweetened almond milk (240 ml)
- 1 apple, skinned and cubed (about 150 g)

- 1/2 tsp ground cinnamon (2.5 ml)
- 1 tbsp chopped walnuts (8 g)
- 1 tbsp maple syrup (optional) (15 ml)
- Fresh apple slices for topping

Directions:

1. Inside your saucepot, blend quinoa, almond milk, cubed apple, and ground cinnamon.
2. Boil, then decrease temp. to low, cover, then simmer for 15 mins or 'til quinoa is cooked.
3. Stir in chopped walnuts and maple syrup if anticipated.
4. Split the porridge into containers and top with fresh apple slices.
5. Present warm.

Per serving: 280 kcal; Fat: 8g; Carbs: 45g; Protein: 8g; Fiber: 6g; Sugar: 12g; Sodium: 100mg; Glycemic Index: 35

---

14. Quinoa Breakfast Bowl

Preparation time: 5 mins

Cooking time: 15 mins

Servings: 2

Ingredients:

- 1 cup quinoa, washed (170 g)
- 2 cups water (480 ml)
- 1 cup fresh berries (e.g., blueberries, strawberries) (150 g)
- 1 tbsp chopped nuts (e.g., almonds, walnuts) (8 g)
- 1 tbsp chia seeds (12 g)
- 1 tsp cinnamon (5 ml)
- 1/2 cup unsweetened almond milk (120 ml)

Directions:

1. Inside your medium saucepan, bring 2 cups of water to a boil.
2. Include washed quinoa to boiling water, decrease temp., cover, then simmer for 15 mins or 'til water is immersed.
3. In serving containers, divide cooked quinoa.
4. Top with fresh berries, chopped nuts, chia seeds, and a sprinkle of cinnamon.
5. Pour a splash of unsweetened almond milk over every container.
6. Stir carefully and relish.

Per serving: 300 kcal; Fat: 8g; Carbs: 48g; Protein: 9g; Fiber: 8g; Sugar: 4g; Sodium: 10mg; Glycemic Index: 35

---

15.   Avocado and Egg Toast

Preparation time: 5 mins

Cooking time: 5 mins

Servings: 2

Ingredients:

- 2 slices whole grain bread, toasted
- 1 ripe avocado, mashed
- 2 eggs, poached or fried
- Salt and pepper as required
- Optional toppings: red pepper flakes, chives, or cherry tomatoes

Directions:

1. Toast the whole grain bread slices.
2. Disperse mashed avocado uniformly over each slice.
3. Top each slice with your poached or fried egg.
4. Flavour using salt and pepper.
5. Optional: include red pepper flakes, chives, or cherry tomatoes for extra flavor.
6. Present instantly.

Per serving: 320 kcal; Fat: 20g; Carbs: 24g; Protein: 14g; Fiber: 8g; Sugar: 2g; Sodium: 250mg; Glycemic Index: 25

---

16.   Tomato Basil Mozzarella Frittata

Preparation time: 10 mins

Cooking time: 15 mins

Servings: 4

Ingredients:

- 6 eggs
- 1 cup cherry tomatoes, halved (150 g)
- 1/2 cup fresh mozzarella, cubed (60 g)
- 1/4 cup fresh basil, chopped (10 g)
- 1 tbsp olive oil (15 ml)
- Salt and pepper as required

Directions:

1. Warm up the oven to 375 deg.F.(190 deg.C.)
2. Inside your container, beat the eggs then flavour using salt and pepper.
3. Warm olive oil in an oven-safe griddle in a middling temp.
4. Include cherry tomatoes to the griddle then cook 'til they start to soften.
5. Pour the whisked eggs over the tomatoes and scatter fresh mozzarella and chopped basil uniformly.

6. Cook on the stovetop for 2-3 mins till the edges set.

7. Transfer the griddle to the warmed up oven then bake for 10-12 mins or 'til the frittata is established.

8. Cut and present warm.

Per serving: 220 kcal; Fat: 16g; Carbs: 6g; Protein: 14g; Fiber: 1g; Sugar: 2g; Sodium: 280mg; Glycemic Index: 15

---

17. Whole Grain Toast with Avocado and Tomato

Preparation time: 5 mins

Cooking time: 5 mins

Servings: 2

Ingredients:

- 4 slices whole grain bread, toasted
- 1 ripe avocado, mashed
- 1 big tomato, sliced
- Salt and pepper as required
- Optional: a sprinkle of chili flakes or herbs for extra flavor

Directions:

1. Toast the whole grain bread slices till golden.
2. Disperse mashed avocado uniformly over each slice.
3. Top with tomato slices then flavour using salt and pepper.
4. Optional: include a sprinkle of chili flakes or herbs for extra flavor.
5. Present instantly.

Per serving: 220 kcal; Fat: 10g; Carbs: 30g; Protein: 7g; Fiber: 8g; Sugar: 3g; Sodium: 180mg; Glycemic Index: 30

---

18. Cauliflower Hash Browns

Preparation time: 15 mins

Cooking time: 15 mins

Servings: 4

Ingredients:

- 4 cups cauliflower rice (about 480 g)
- 1/4 cup almond flour (30 g)
- 2 eggs, whisked
- 1/4 cup grated Parmesan cheese (25 g)
- 1 tsp garlic powder (5 ml)

- 1 tsp onion powder (5 ml)
- Salt and pepper as required
- Cooking spray

Directions:

1. Warm up the oven to 400 deg.F.(200 deg.C.) after that, prepare your baking sheet by lining it with parchment paper.
2. Inside your big container, blend cauliflower rice, almond flour, whisked eggs, Parmesan cheese, garlic powder, onion powder, salt, and pepper.
3. Mix till well blended.
4. Form the solution into hash brown shapes and put them on the prepared baking sheet.
5. Use cooking sprinkle on top.
6. Bake for 15 mins, then flip then bake for an extra 10-15 mins or 'til golden brown and crispy.
7. Present hot.

Per serving: 120 kcal; Fat: 8g; Carbs: 8g; Protein: 6g; Fiber: 3g; Sugar: 2g; Sodium: 160mg; Glycemic Index: 20

---

19.   Peanut Butter Banana Smoothie

Preparation time: 5 mins

Cooking time: 0 mins

Servings: 2

Ingredients:

- 2 ripe bananas, skinned and frozen
- 2 tbsps natural peanut butter (30 ml)
- 1 cup unsweetened almond milk (240 ml)
- 1/2 cup Greek yogurt (120 g)
- 1 tsp honey (optional) (5 ml)
- Ice cubes (optional)

Directions:

1. Inside a mixer, blend frozen bananas, peanut butter, almond milk, Greek yogurt, and honey (if using).
2. Blend till smooth and creamy.
3. If desired, include ice cubes then blend again till well blended.
4. Pour into glasses and present instantly.

Per serving: 300 kcal; Fat: 16g; Carbs: 30g; Protein: 10g; Fiber: 4g; Sugar: 15g; Sodium: 180mg; Glycemic Index: 35

---

20. Mexican Breakfast Casserole

Preparation time: 20 mins

Cooking time: 30 mins

Servings: 6

Ingredients:

- 1 lb. ground turkey or chicken (454 g)
- 1 onion, cubed (150 g)
- 1 bell pepper, cubed (150 g)
- 1 cup black beans, drained and washed (240 g)
- 1 cup corn kernels (150 g)
- 1 tsp chili powder (5 ml)
- 1/2 tsp cumin (2.5 ml)
- Salt and pepper as required
- 8 big eggs
- 1/2 cup milk (almond or regular) (120 ml)
- 1 cup torn cheddar cheese (120 g)
- Fresh cilantro for garnish (optional)
- Salsa for serving

Directions:

1. Warm up the oven to 375 deg.F.(190 deg.C.) then oil your baking dish.
2. Inside your griddle, cook ground turkey or chicken till browned.
3. Include cubed onion and bell pepper, cooking till softened.
4. Stir in black beans, corn, chili powder, cumin, salt, and pepper. Cook for an extra 2-3 mins.
5. Inside your container, whisk together eggs and milk.
6. Disperse the turkey solution uniformly in the arranged baking dish.
7. Pour egg solution over the turkey solution.
8. sprinkle torn cheddar cheese on top.
9. Bake for 25-30 mins or 'til the eggs are set.
10. Decorate with fresh cilantro if anticipated and present with salsa.

Per serving: 320 kcal; Fat: 18g; Carbs: 18g; Protein: 22g; Fiber: 4g; Sugar: 4g; Sodium: 420mg; Glycemic Index: 25

CHAPTER 3: Lunch Recipes

1.   Grilled Chicken Salad with Vinaigrette

Preparation time: 15 mins

Cooking time: 15 mins

Servings: 4

Ingredients:

- 1 lb. boneless, skinless chicken breasts (454 g)
- 6 cups mixed salad greens (e.g., spinach, arugula, and romaine) (180 g)
- 1 cup cherry tomatoes, halved (150 g)
- 1 cucumber, sliced
- 1/4 cup red onion, finely sliced (40 g)
- 1/4 cup feta cheese, crumbled (optional) (30 g)

Vinaigrette:

- 3 tbsps olive oil (45 ml)
- 2 tbsps balsamic vinegar (30 ml)
- 1 tsp Dijon mustard (5 ml)
- Salt and pepper as required

Directions:

1. Warm up the grill to med-high temp.
2. Flavour chicken breasts using salt and pepper.
3. Grill chicken for around 6-7 mins on all sides or 'til fully cooked.
4. Inside your big container, blend salad greens, cherry tomatoes, cucumber, red onion, and feta cheese.
5. Inside your small container, whisk together olive oil, salt, balsamic vinegar, Dijon mustard, and pepper to create the vinaigrette.
6. Slice grilled chicken and place on top of the salad.
7. sprinkle using vinaigrette over the salad then shake carefully to blend.
8. Present instantly.

Per serving: 300 kcal; Fat: 15g; Carbs: 10g; Protein: 30g; Fiber: 3g; Sugar: 5g; Sodium: 200mg; Glycemic Index: 20

2.   Turkey Lettuce Wraps

Preparation time: 20 mins

Cooking time: 10 mins

Servings: 4

Ingredients:

- 1 lb. ground turkey (454 g)
- 1 tbsp olive oil (15 ml)
- 1 onion, finely chopped (150 g)
- 2 pieces garlic, crushed
- 1 red bell pepper, cubed (150 g)
- 1 zucchini, grated (200 g)
- 1 tsp ground cumin (5 ml)
- 1 tsp chili powder (5 ml)
- Salt and pepper as required
- Iceberg or butter lettuce leaves for wrapping

Directions:

1. Inside your griddle, warm olive oil in a middling temp.
2. Include chopped onion, garlic, then cook 'til softened.
3. Include ground turkey then cook 'til browned.
4. Stir in bell pepper, grated zucchini, cumin, chili powder, salt, and pepper. Cook for an extra 5 mins.
5. Spoon the turkey solution into lettuce leaves.
6. Present instantly.

Per serving: 250 kcal; Fat: 12g; Carbs: 10g; Protein: 25g; Fiber: 3g; Sugar: 4g; Sodium: 150mg; Glycemic Index: 30

---

3.   Quinoa and Black Bean Stuffed Peppers

Preparation time: 15 mins

Cooking time: 30 mins

Servings: 4

Ingredients:

- 4 bell peppers, halved and seeds removed
- 1 cup quinoa, cooked (185 g)
- 1 tin (15 oz) black beans, drained and washed (425 g)
- 1 cup corn kernels (fresh or frozen) (150 g)
- 1 cup cubed tomatoes (150 g)
- 1 tsp ground cumin (5 ml)
- 1 tsp chili powder (5 ml)

- Salt and pepper as required
- 1/2 cup torn low-fat cheese (optional) (60 g)

Directions:

1. Warm up the oven to 375 deg.F.(190 deg.C.)
2. Inside your container, blend cooked quinoa, black beans, corn, cubed tomatoes, cumin, chili powder, salt, and pepper.
3. Stuff each bell pepper half with your quinoa and black bean solution.
4. Put filled peppers in your baking dish.
5. If desired, sprinkle torn cheese on top.
6. Bake for 25-30 mins or 'til peppers are soft.
7. Present hot.

Per serving: 280 kcal; Fat: 5g; Carbs: 50g; Protein: 12g; Fiber: 10g; Sugar: 6g; Sodium: 200mg; Glycemic Index: 40

---

4.   Mediterranean Chickpea Salad

Preparation time: 15 mins

Cooking time: 0 mins

Servings: 4

Ingredients:

- 2 tins (15 oz each) chickpeas, drained and washed (850 g)
- 1 cucumber, cubed
- 1 cup cherry tomatoes, halved (150 g)
- 1/2 red onion, finely chopped (40 g)
- 1/2 cup Kalamata olives, sliced (75 g)
- 1/2 cup crumbled feta cheese (60 g)
- 3 tbsps extra-virgin olive oil (45 ml)
- 2 tbsps red wine vinegar (30 ml)
- 1 tsp dried oregano (5 ml)
- Salt and pepper as required
- Fresh parsley for garnish

Directions:

1. Inside your big container, blend chickpeas, cucumber, cherry tomatoes, red onion, olives, and feta cheese.
2. Inside your small container, whisk together olive oil, salt, red wine vinegar, dried oregano, and pepper.
3. Spread the coating across the salad and set it aside. then shake carefully to cover.
4. Decorate with fresh parsley as a finishing touch.

5. Present chilled.

Per serving: 320 kcal; Fat: 18g; Carbs: 32g; Protein: 10g; Fiber: 8g; Sugar: 5g; Sodium: 450mg; Glycemic Index: 30

---

5.   Salmon and Asparagus Foil Packets

Preparation time: 10 mins

Cooking time: 20 mins

Servings: 2

Ingredients:

- 2 salmon fillets
- 1 bunch asparagus, clipped (about 250 g)
- 1 lemon, sliced
- 2 tbsp olive oil (30 ml)
- 2 pieces garlic, crushed
- 1 tsp dried dill (5 ml)
- Salt and pepper as required

Directions:

1. Warm up the oven to 400 deg.F.(200 deg.C.)
2. Put each salmon fillet on your big piece of foil.
3. Organize asparagus around the salmon fillets.
4. sprinkle olive oil over the salmon and asparagus.
5. sprinkle crushed garlic, dried dill, salt, and pepper over the top.
6. Place lemon slices on each salmon fillet.
7. Seal the foil packets firmly and put them on your baking sheet.
8. Bake for 18-20 mins or 'til salmon is fully cooked.
9. Present hot.

Per serving: 400 kcal; Fat: 25g; Carbs: 12g; Protein: 30g; Fiber: 5g; Sugar: 3g; Sodium: 150mg; Glycemic Index: 20

---

6.   Spinach and Feta Turkey Burger

Preparation time: 15 mins

Cooking time: 15 mins

Servings: 4

Ingredients:

- 1 lb. ground turkey (454 g)
- 1 cup fresh spinach, chopped (30 g)

- 1/2 cup crumbled feta cheese (60 g)
- 1/4 cup red onion, finely chopped (40 g)
- 1 tsp dried oregano (5 ml)
- Salt and pepper as required
- Whole wheat burger buns
- Lettuce and tomato slices for garnish

Directions:

1. Inside your container, blend ground turkey, chopped spinach, feta cheese, red onion, dried oregano, salt, and pepper.
2. Form the solution into 4 burger patties.
3. Grill or cook in a griddle in a middling temp. for around 6-7 mins on all sides or 'til fully cooked.
4. Toast whole wheat burger buns.
5. Place a turkey burger on each bun then garnish with lettuce and tomato slices.
6. Present hot.

Per serving: 280 kcal; Fat: 15g; Carbs: 15g; Protein: 20g; Fiber: 3g; Sugar: 2g; Sodium: 300mg; Glycemic Index: 25

---

7. Cauliflower Rice Stir-Fry with Tofu

Preparation time: 20 mins

Cooking time: 15 mins

Servings: 4

Ingredients:

- 1 block firm tofu, pressed and cubed (about 400 g)
- 4 cups cauliflower rice (store-bought or homemade) (600 g)
- 1 cup broccoli florets (150 g)
- 1 bell pepper, finely sliced (about 150 g)
- 2 carrots, julienned (about 100 g)
- 3 green onions, chopped
- 2 pieces garlic, crushed
- 3 tbsps low-sodium soy sauce (45 ml)
- 1 tbsp sesame oil (15 ml)
- 1 tsp ginger, grated (5 ml)
- Sesame seeds for garnish

Directions:

1. Inside your big griddle or wok, warm sesame oil in a med-high temp.
2. Include cubed tofu then cook 'til golden brown on all sides.
3. Push tofu to one side of the pan and include garlic and ginger to the other side. Sauté briefly.

4. Include broccoli, bell pepper, carrots, and cauliflower rice to the pan. Cook 'til vegetables are soft-crisp.

5. Stir in soy sauce and green onions. Cook for an extra 2-3 mins.

6. Decorate with sesame seeds.

7. Present hot.

Per serving: 250 kcal; Fat: 12g; Carbs: 20g; Protein: 15g; Fiber: 8g; Sugar: 5g; Sodium: 500mg; Glycemic Index: 20

---

8. Turkey and Avocado Wrap

Preparation time: 10 mins

Cooking time: 0 mins

Servings: 2

Ingredients:

- 8 oz sliced turkey breast (227 g)
- 1 avocado, sliced
- 1 cup mixed salad greens (30 g)
- 1/4 cup cherry tomatoes, halved (37.5 g)
- 2 whole wheat wraps

Greek Yogurt Dressing:

- 1/2 cup Greek yogurt (120 g)
- 1 tbsp lime juice (15 ml)
- 1 tsp honey (5 ml)
- Salt and pepper as required

Directions:

1. Inside your small container, blend together Greek yogurt, lime juice, honey, salt, and pepper to create the dressing.

2. Lay out the whole wheat wraps and uniformly distribute turkey slices, avocado, mixed salad greens, and cherry tomatoes.

3. sprinkle using Greek yogurt dressing over the components.

4. Fold the sides of the wrap then roll firmly.

5. Slice in half and present.

Per serving: 400 kcal; Fat: 15g; Carbs: 45g; Protein: 20g; Fiber: 8g; Sugar: 5g; Sodium: 500mg; Glycemic Index: 25

---

9. Shrimp and Vegetable Skewers

Preparation time: 20 mins

Cooking time: 10 mins

Servings: 4

Ingredients:

- 1 lb. big shrimp, skinned and deveined (454 g)
- 1 zucchini, sliced (about 200 g)
- 1 bell pepper, cut into chunks (about 150 g)
- 1 red onion, cut into chunks (about 150 g)
- Cherry tomatoes (about 200 g)
- 2 tbsp olive oil (30 ml)
- 1 tsp smoked paprika (5 ml)
- 1 tsp garlic powder (5 ml)
- Salt and pepper as required
- Lemon wedges for serving

Directions:

1. Warm up the grill pan to med-high temp.
2. Inside your container, blend shrimp, zucchini, bell pepper, red onion, and cherry tomatoes.
3. Inside your small container, blend together olive oil, smoked paprika, garlic powder, salt, and pepper.
4. Thread shrimp and vegetables onto skewers, alternating between each.
5. Brush skewers with the olive oil solution.
6. Grill for 3-4 mins on all sides or 'til shrimp is opaque and vegetables are soft.
7. Present with lemon wedges.

Per serving: 250 kcal; Fat: 10g; Carbs: 15g; Protein: 25g; Fiber: 4g; Sugar: 6g; Sodium: 300mg; Glycemic Index: 20

---

10. Tomato Basil Chicken Wrap

Preparation time: 15 mins

Cooking time: 15 mins

Servings: 2

Ingredients:

- 2 boneless, skinless chicken breasts (about 454 g)
- 1 tbsp olive oil (15 ml)
- Salt and pepper as required
- 2 whole wheat wraps
- 1 cup cherry tomatoes, halved (150 g)

- 1/2 cup fresh basil leaves (about 15 g)
- 1/4 cup balsamic glaze (60 ml)

Directions:

1. Flavour chicken breasts using salt and pepper.
2. Inside your griddle, warm olive oil in a med-high temp.
3. Cook your chicken breasts for 6-7 mins on all sides or 'til fully cooked.
4. Slice the cooked chicken into strips.
5. Lay out the whole wheat wraps and uniformly distribute chicken strips, cherry tomatoes, and fresh basil leaves.
6. sprinkle balsamic glaze over the components.
7. Fold the sides of the wrap then roll firmly.
8. Slice in half and present.

Per serving: 350 kcal; Fat: 10g; Carbs: 40g; Protein: 25g; Fiber: 8g; Sugar: 10g; Sodium: 400mg; Glycemic Index: 30

---

11.   Broccoli and Chicken Quiche

Preparation time: 20 mins

Cooking time: 40 mins

Servings: 6

Ingredients:

- 1 pre-made pie crust (whole wheat if available)
- 1 cup cooked chicken breast, torn (about 150 g)
- 1 cup broccoli florets, steamed and chopped (about 150 g)
- 1/2 cup cherry tomatoes, halved (75 g)
- 1/2 cup feta cheese, crumbled (60 g)
- 4 big eggs
- 1 cup low-fat milk (240 ml)
- Salt and pepper as required
- 1/2 tsp dried thyme (2.5 ml)

Directions:

1. Warm up the oven to 375 deg.F.(190 deg.C.)
2. Place pie crust in a pie dish then crimp the edges.
3. Inside your container, blend together chicken, broccoli, cherry tomatoes, and feta cheese. Disperse uniformly in the pie crust.
4. Inside a distinct container, whisk together eggs, milk, salt, pepper, and dried thyme.
5. Pour egg solution over the chicken and vegetable filling.
6. Bake for 35-40 mins or 'til the center is set and the top is golden brown.

7. Allow it to rest for a couple of mins prior to slicing.

Per serving: 300 kcal; Fat: 15g; Carbs: 25g; Protein: 18g; Fiber: 2g; Sugar: 3g; Sodium: 400mg; Glycemic Index: 25

---

12.   Cucumber and Radish Salad with Feta

Preparation time: 10 mins

Cooking time: 0 mins

Servings: 4

Ingredients:

- 2 cucumbers, finely sliced
- 1 bunch radishes, finely sliced
- 1/2 cup crumbled feta cheese (60 g)
- 1/4 cup red onion, finely sliced (40 g)
- 2 tbsps olive oil (30 ml)
- 1 tbsp red wine vinegar (15 ml)
- 1 tsp Dijon mustard (5 ml)
- Salt and pepper as required
- Fresh dill for garnish (optional)

Directions:

1. Inside your big container, blend sliced cucumbers, radishes, feta cheese, and red onion.
2. Inside your small container, whisk together salt, olive oil, red wine vinegar, Dijon mustard, and pepper.
3. Spread the coating across the salad and set it aside. then shake carefully to cover.
4. Decorate with fresh dill if anticipated.
5. Present chilled.

Per serving: 180 kcal; Fat: 14g; Carbs: 10g; Protein: 5g; Fiber: 2g; Sugar: 4g; Sodium: 250mg; Glycemic Index: 20

---

13.   Minestrone Soup with Whole Wheat Pasta

Preparation time: 15 mins

Cooking time: 30 mins

Servings: 6

Ingredients:

- 1 cup whole wheat pasta, uncooked (about 90 g)
- 1 tbsp olive oil (15 ml)
- 1 onion, cubed (150 g)

- 2 carrots, cubed (120 g)
- 2 celery stalks, cubed (80 g)
- 3 pieces garlic, crushed
- 1 tin (15 oz) cubed tomatoes, undrained (425 g)
- 6 cups low-sodium vegetable broth (1.44 liters)
- 1 tin (15 oz) kidney beans, drained and washed (425 g)
- 1 zucchini, cubed (200 g)
- 1 cup green beans, chopped (150 g)
- 1 tsp dried oregano (5 ml)
- 1 tsp dried basil (5 ml)
- Salt and pepper as required
- Grated Parmesan cheese for garnish (optional)

Directions:

1. Cook whole wheat pasta using the package guidelines. Drain then put away.
2. Inside your big pot, warm olive oil in a middling temp.
3. Include onion, carrots, celery, and garlic. Sauté till vegetables are softened.
4. Stir in cubed tomatoes, vegetable broth, kidney beans, zucchini, green beans, oregano, basil, salt, and pepper.
5. Boil, then decrease temp. then simmer for 20-25 mins.
6. Include cooked pasta to the pot then simmer for an extra 5 mins.
7. You might have to make changes to the seasoning.
8. Present hot, garnished using grated Parmesan cheese if anticipated.

Per serving: 280 kcal; Fat: 5g; Carbs: 50g; Protein: 12g; Fiber: 10g; Sugar: 8g; Sodium: 500mg; Glycemic Index: 35

---

14. Grilled Veggie and Hummus Wrap

Preparation time: 15 mins

Cooking time: 10 mins

Servings: 2

Ingredients:

- 1 zucchini, sliced (about 200 g)
- 1 red bell pepper, sliced (about 150 g)
- 1 yellow bell pepper, sliced (about 150 g)
- 1 small eggplant, sliced (about 300 g)
- 2 whole wheat wraps
- 1/2 cup hummus (low-fat if available) (120 g)
- Fresh spinach leaves

- Salt and pepper as required

Directions:

1. Warm up the grill pan to med-high temp.
2. Grill zucchini, red bell pepper, yellow bell pepper, and eggplant slices till soft.
3. Lay out the whole wheat wraps and spread a generous layer of hummus on each.
4. Place grilled vegetables and fresh spinach leaves on the wraps.
5. Flavour using salt and pepper as required.
6. Fold the sides of the wrap then roll firmly.
7. Slice in half and present.

Per serving: 350 kcal; Fat: 12g; Carbs: 50g; Protein: 12g; Fiber: 12g; Sugar: 8g; Sodium: 400mg; Glycemic Index: 25

---

15. Pesto Zoodles with Cherry Tomatoes

Preparation time: 15 mins

Cooking time: 5 mins

Servings: 2

Ingredients:

- 4 medium zucchinis, spiralized into zoodles (about 800 g)
- 1 cup cherry tomatoes, halved (150 g)
- 1/4 cup pesto sauce (store-bought or homemade) (60 ml)
- 2 tbsp grated Parmesan cheese (10 g)
- Salt and pepper as required
- Fresh basil leaves for garnish

Directions:

1. Spiralize the zucchinis into zoodles using a spiralizer.
2. Inside your big pan, heat a bit of olive oil in a middling temp.
3. Include zoodles to the pan and sauté for 2-3 mins till just soft.
4. Shake in cherry tomatoes then cook for an extra 2 mins.
5. Stir in pesto sauce then cook 'til everything is well covered.
6. Flavour using salt and pepper as required.
7. Present in containers, sprinkle with grated Parmesan cheese, then garnish with fresh basil leaves.

Per serving: 200 kcal; Fat: 12g; Carbs: 15g; Protein: 8g; Fiber: 5g; Sugar: 8g; Sodium: 300mg; Glycemic Index: 15

16.   Tuna Salad Lettuce Wraps

Preparation time: 10 mins

Cooking time: 0 mins

Servings: 2

Ingredients:

- 2 tins (5 oz each) tuna in water, drained (total 284 g)
- 1/4 cup Greek yogurt (60 g)
- 2 tbsp mayonnaise (low-fat if available) (30 ml)
- 1 celery stalk, finely chopped (40 g)
- 1/4 red onion, finely chopped (40 g)
- 1 tbsp Dijon mustard (15 ml)
- Salt and pepper as required
- Butter lettuce leaves for wrapping
- Tomato slices for garnish

Directions:

1. Inside your container, blend tuna, salt, Greek yogurt, mayonnaise, celery, red onion, Dijon mustard, and pepper.
2. Mix till well blended.
3. Spoon tuna salad onto butter lettuce leaves.
4. Decorate with tomato slices.
5. Present instantly.

Per serving: 250 kcal; Fat: 10g; Carbs: 5g; Protein: 30g; Fiber: 2g; Sugar: 2g; Sodium: 400mg; Glycemic Index: 10

---

17.   Chicken and Vegetable Kabobs

Preparation time: 20 mins

Cooking time: 15 mins

Servings: 4

Ingredients:

- 1 lb. boneless, skinless chicken breast, cut into cubes (454 g)
- 1 zucchini, sliced (about 200 g)
- 1 bell pepper, cut into chunks (about 150 g)
- 1 red onion, cut into chunks (about 150 g)
- Cherry tomatoes (about 200 g)
- 2 tbsps olive oil (30 ml)
- 2 tbsps lemon juice (30 ml)
- 1 tsp dried oregano (5 ml)

- 1 tsp garlic powder (5 ml)
- Salt and pepper as required
- Wooden or metal skewers

Directions:

1. If using wooden skewers, that is soak them in water for 30 mins to avoid burning.
2. Inside your container, mix olive oil, salt, lemon juice, dried oregano, garlic powder, and pepper to create the marinade.
3. Thread chicken cubes, zucchini, bell pepper, red onion, and cherry tomatoes into your skewers.
4. Brush the kabobs with the marinade.
5. Warm up the grill pan to med-high temp.
6. Grill the kabobs for 12-15 mins, turning irregularly, till the chicken is fully cooked.
7. Present hot.

Per serving: 280 kcal; Fat: 12g; Carbs: 10g; Protein: 30g; Fiber: 3g; Sugar: 5g; Sodium: 350mg; Glycemic Index: 15

18.   Caprese Salad with Balsamic Glaze

Preparation time: 10 mins

Cooking time: 0 mins

Servings: 2

Ingredients:

- 2 big tomatoes, sliced
- 1 ball fresh mozzarella, sliced (approximately 125 g)
- Fresh basil leaves
- Balsamic glaze (as desired)
- Extra-virgin olive oil (as desired)
- Salt and pepper as required

Directions:

1. Organize tomato and mozzarella slices interchangeably on a serving plate.
2. You should sandwich some fresh basil leaves among the pieces of tomato and mozzarella.
3. sprinkle with balsamic glaze and olive oil.
4. sprinkle using salt and pepper as required.
5. Present instantly as a refreshing salad.

Per serving: 250 kcal; Fat: 18g; Carbs: 10g; Protein: 12g; Fiber: 2g; Sugar: 5g; Sodium: 350mg; Glycemic Index: 20

19.   Eggplant and Chickpea Stew

Preparation time: 15 mins

Cooking time: 30 mins

Servings: 4

Ingredients:

- 1 big eggplant, cubed (about 500 g)
- 1 tin (15 oz) chickpeas, drained and washed (425 g)
- 1 onion, chopped (150 g)
- 2 pieces garlic, crushed
- 1 tin (14 oz) cubed tomatoes (400 g)
- 1 cup vegetable broth (240 ml)
- 1 tsp ground cumin (5 ml)
- 1 tsp smoked paprika (5 ml)
- Salt and pepper as required
- Fresh parsley for garnish

Directions:

1. Inside your big pot, sauté onion and garlic till softened.
2. Include cubed eggplant then cook for 5 mins.
3. Stir in chickpeas, cubed tomatoes, vegetable broth, ground cumin, smoked paprika, salt, and pepper.
4. Boil, then decrease temp. Then simmer for 20-25 mins or 'til eggplant is soft.
5. You might have to make changes to the seasoning.
6. Decorate with fresh parsley as a finishing touch.
7. Present hot.

Per serving: 220 kcal; Fat: 3g; Carbs: 40g; Protein: 10g; Fiber: 10g; Sugar: 8g; Sodium: 400mg; Glycemic Index: 25

---

20.   Turkey and Spinach Stuffed Mushrooms

Preparation time: 20 mins

Cooking time: 15 mins

Servings: 4

Ingredients:

- 16 big mushrooms, stems removed
- 1/2 lb. ground turkey (227 g)
- 1 cup fresh spinach, chopped (30 g)
- 1/4 cup onion, finely chopped (40 g)
- 2 pieces garlic, crushed

- 1/4 cup feta cheese, crumbled (30 g)
- 1 tsp dried oregano (5 ml)
- Salt and pepper as required
- Olive oil for drizzling (as desired)

Directions:

1. Warm up the oven to 375 deg.F.(190 deg.C.)
2. Inside your griddle, cook ground turkey till browned.
3. Include chopped spinach, onion, and garlic to the griddle. Cook 'til spinach is wilted.
4. Stir in feta cheese, dried oregano, salt, and pepper.
5. Fill each mushroom cap with the turkey and spinach solution.
6. sprinkle with a small amount of olive oil.
7. Place filled mushrooms on your baking sheet then bake for 15 mins or 'til mushrooms are soft.
8. Present warm.

Per serving: 180 kcal; Fat: 8g; Carbs: 10g; Protein: 18g; Fiber: 3g; Sugar: 3g; Sodium: 250mg; Glycemic Index: 15

CHAPTER 4: Dinner Recipes

1.   Baked Lemon Herb Chicken

Preparation time: 15 mins

Cooking time: 30 mins

Servings: 4

Ingredients:

- 4 boneless, skinless chicken breasts (about 680 g)
- Zest and juice of 1 lemon (about 1 tbsp zest and 2-3 tbsp juice)
- 2 tbsp olive oil (30 ml)
- 2 pieces garlic, crushed
- 1 tsp dried oregano (5 ml)
- 1 tsp dried thyme (5 ml)
- Salt and pepper as required
- Fresh parsley for garnish

Directions:

1. Warm up the oven to 400 deg.F.(200 deg.C.)
2. Inside your container, blend together lemon zest, lemon juice, olive oil, crushed garlic, dried oregano, dried thyme, salt, and pepper.
3. Place chicken breasts in your baking dish then pour the lemon herb solution over them.
4. Bake for 25-30 mins or 'til the chicken is fully cooked.
5. Decorate with fresh parsley as a finishing touch prior to presenting.

Per serving: 250 kcal; Fat: 12g; Carbs: 2g; Protein: 30g; Fiber: 1g; Sugar: 1g; Sodium: 350mg; Glycemic Index: 5

---

2.   Quinoa-Stuffed Bell Peppers

Preparation time: 20 mins

Cooking time: 30 mins

Servings: 4

Ingredients:

- 4 bell peppers, divided and seeds taken out
- 1 cup (190g) quinoa, cooked
- 1 tin (15 oz or 425g) black beans, drained and rinsed
- 1 cup (150g) corn kernels (fresh or frozen)
- 1 cup (150g) cherry tomatoes, cubed

- 1/2 cup (75g) red onion, finely chopped
- 1 tsp (5 ml) ground cumin
- 1 tsp (5 ml) chili powder
- Salt and pepper as required
- 1 cup (100g) torn cheddar cheese
- Fresh cilantro for garnish

Directions:
1. Warm up the oven to 375 deg.F.(190 deg.C.)
2. Inside your container, blend together cooked quinoa, black beans, corn, cherry tomatoes, red onion, ground cumin, chili powder, salt, and pepper.
3. Stuff each bell pepper half utilizing the quinoa solution.
4. Top each filled pepper with torn cheddar cheese.
5. Bake for 25-30 mins or 'til the peppers are soft and the cheese is dissolved.
6. Decorate with fresh cilantro prior to presenting.

Per serving: 350 kcal; Fat: 10g; Carbs: 50g; Protein: 15g; Fiber: 10g; Sugar: 8g; Sodium: 300mg; Glycemic Index: 15

---

3.   Garlic Parmesan Baked Cod

Preparation time: 10 mins

Cooking time: 15 mins

Servings: 4

Ingredients:
- 4 cod fillets
- 2 tbsps (30 ml) olive oil
- 4 pieces garlic, crushed
- 1/2 cup (50g) grated Parmesan cheese
- 1 tsp (5 ml) dried oregano
- Salt and pepper as required
- Fresh parsley for garnish
- Lemon wedges for serving

Directions:
1. Warm up the oven to 400 deg.F.(200 deg.C.)
2. Place cod fillets in your baking dish.
3. Inside your small container, blend together olive oil, crushed garlic, grated Parmesan cheese, dried oregano, salt, and pepper.
4. Disperse the Parmesan solution over the cod fillets.
5. Bake for 12-15 mins or 'til the fish is opaque and flakes simply.

6. Decorate with fresh parsley as a finishing touch and present with lemon wedges.

Per serving: 220 kcal; Fat: 10g; Carbs: 2g; Protein: 30g; Fiber: 0g; Sugar: 0g; Sodium: 300mg; Glycemic Index: 5

---

4.   Cauliflower and Lentil Curry

Preparation time: 15 mins

Cooking time: 25 mins

Servings: 6

Ingredients:

- 1 cup (200g) dry lentils, washed and drained
- 1 head cauliflower, cut into florets
- 1 tin (14 oz or 400g) cubed tomatoes
- 1 onion, finely chopped
- 3 pieces garlic, crushed
- 1 tbsp (15 ml) curry powder
- 1 tsp (5 ml) ground cumin
- 1 tsp (5 ml) ground coriander
- 1/2 tsp (2.5 ml) turmeric
- 1 tin (14 oz or 400g) coconut milk
- Salt and pepper as required
- Fresh cilantro for garnish
- Cooked brown rice for serving

Directions:

1. Inside your big pot, blend lentils, cauliflower, cubed tomatoes, chopped onion, crushed garlic, curry powder, cumin, coriander, turmeric, coconut milk, salt, and pepper.
2. Boil, then decrease temp. Then simmer for 20-25 mins or 'til lentils and cauliflower are soft.
3. You might have to make changes to the seasoning.
4. Present over cooked brown rice then garnish with fresh cilantro.

Per serving: 320 kcal; Fat: 12g; Carbs: 40g; Protein: 15g; Fiber: 15g; Sugar: 5g; Sodium: 350mg; Glycemic Index: 30

---

5.   Greek Quinoa Salad

Preparation time: 15 mins

Cooking time: 15 mins (for quinoa)

Servings: 4

Ingredients:

- 1 cup (190g) quinoa, washed
- 2 cups (480 ml) water
- 1 cucumber, cubed
- 1 cup (150g) cherry tomatoes, halved
- 1/2 cup (90g) Kalamata olives, sliced
- 1/2 cup (75g) crumbled feta cheese
- 1/4 cup (40g) red onion, finely chopped
- 1/4 cup (15g) fresh parsley, chopped

Greek Dressing:
- 3 tbsps (45 ml) extra-virgin olive oil
- 2 tbsps (30 ml) red wine vinegar
- 1 tsp (5 ml) dried oregano
- Salt and pepper as required

Directions:
1. Cook quinoa using the package guidelines.
2. Inside your big container, blend cooked quinoa, cucumber, cherry tomatoes, olives, feta cheese, red onion, and parsley.
3. Inside your small container, whisk together salt, olive oil, red wine vinegar, dried oregano, and pepper to create the dressing.
4. Spread the coating across the salad and set it aside. then shake carefully to blend.
5. Present chilled.

Per serving: 300 kcal; Fat: 15g; Carbs: 35g; Protein: 8g; Fiber: 5g; Sugar: 3g; Sodium: 400mg; Glycemic Index: 30

---

6. Grilled Salmon with Dill Sauce

Preparation time: 15 mins

Cooking time: 10 mins

Servings: 4

Ingredients:

For the Salmon:
- 4 salmon fillets
- 2 tbsp (30 ml) olive oil
- Salt and pepper as required
- 2 tbsp (8g) fresh dill, chopped

Dill Sauce:
- 1/2 cup (120g) Greek yogurt
- 2 tbsp (8g) fresh dill, chopped

- 1 tbsp (15 ml) Dijon mustard
- 1 tbsp (15 ml) lemon juice
- Salt and pepper as required

Directions:

1. Warm up the grill to med-high temp.
2. Rub salmon fillets with olive oil then flavour with salt, pepper, and chopped dill.
3. Grill salmon for 4-5 mins on all sides or 'til fully cooked.
4. Inside your small container, blend together salt, Greek yogurt, dill, Dijon mustard, lemon juice, and pepper to make the sauce.
5. Present grilled salmon with dill sauce on the side.

Per serving: 300 kcal; Fat: 15g; Carbs: 3g; Protein: 35g; Fiber: 1g; Sugar: 2g; Sodium: 350mg; Glycemic Index: 5

---

7. Zucchini Noodles with Pesto and Cherry Tomatoes

Preparation time: 20 mins

Cooking time: 5 mins

Servings: 2

Ingredients:

For the Zucchini Noodles:

- 4 medium zucchinis, spiralized into noodles
- 1 cup (150g) cherry tomatoes, halved
- 1/4 cup (30g) pine nuts, toasted
- 1/2 cup fresh basil leaves
- 1/4 cup (25g) grated Parmesan cheese
- 2 tbsps (30 ml) olive oil
- Salt and pepper as required

Pesto Sauce:

- 2 cups fresh basil leaves
- 1/2 cup (50g) grated Parmesan cheese
- 1/3 cup (45g) pine nuts
- 2 pieces garlic, crushed
- 1/2 cup (120 ml) extra-virgin olive oil
- Salt and pepper as required
-

Directions:

1. Inside a blending container, blend fresh basil, grated Parmesan, pine nuts, and crushed garlic for the pesto sauce. Pulse till finely chopped.

2. With your processor running, slowly pour in the olive oil 'til the pesto reaches a smooth consistency. Flavour using salt and pepper.
3. Inside your big pan, sauté zucchini noodles for 3-4 mins till just soft.
4. Shake zucchini noodles with pesto sauce, cherry tomatoes, toasted pine nuts, and grated Parmesan.
5. Present warm.

Per serving: 350 kcal; Fat: 30g; Carbs: 10g; Protein: 10g; Fiber: 4g; Sugar: 5g; Sodium: 300mg; Glycemic Index: 10

---

8.   Lemon Garlic Shrimp Skewers

Preparation time: 15 mins

Cooking time: 6 mins

Servings: 4

Ingredients:

- 1 lb. (450g) large shrimp, peeled and deveined
- 2 tbsp (30 ml) olive oil
- Zest and juice of 1 lemon
- 3 pieces garlic, crushed
- 1 tsp (5 ml) dried oregano
- Salt and pepper as required
- Wooden or metal skewers

Directions:

1. Inside your container, blend together olive oil, lemon zest, lemon juice, crushed garlic, dried oregano, salt, and pepper.
2. Thread shrimp on skewers, then brush with the lemon-garlic marinade.
3. Warm up the grill pan to med-high temp.
4. Grill shrimp skewers for a total of 3 mins on all sides or 'til shrimp is opaque.
5. Present hot.

Per serving: 200 kcal; Fat: 10g; Carbs: 2g; Protein: 25g; Fiber: 0g; Sugar: 1g; Sodium: 300mg; Glycemic Index: 5

---

9.   Chicken and Broccoli Casserole

Preparation time: 20 mins

Cooking time: 30 mins

Servings: 6

Ingredients:

- 2 lbs. (900g) boneless, skinless chicken breasts, cooked and shredded

- 4 cups (about 300g) broccoli florets, steamed
- 2 cups (370g) brown rice, cooked
- 1 cup (240g) plain Greek yogurt
- 1 cup (240 ml) low-sodium chicken broth
- 1 cup (100g) torn cheddar cheese
- 1/4 cup (25g) grated Parmesan cheese
- 2 pieces garlic, crushed
- 1 tsp (5 ml) onion powder
- Salt and pepper as required

Directions:

1. Warm up the oven to 375 deg.F.(190 deg.C.)
2. Inside your big container, blend torn chicken, steamed broccoli, cooked brown rice, Greek yogurt, chicken broth, crushed garlic, onion powder, salt, and pepper.
3. Transfer solution to an oiled casserole dish.
4. Top with torn cheddar and grated Parmesan cheese.
5. Bake for 25-30 mins or 'til the casserole is fully heated and the cheese is dissolved and bubbly.
6. Allow it to rest for a couple of mins prior to presenting.

Per serving: 400 kcal; Fat: 15g; Carbs: 35g; Protein: 30g; Fiber: 5g; Sugar: 2g; Sodium: 450mg; Glycemic Index: 35

---

10. Spinach and Feta Stuffed Chicken Breast

Preparation time: 15 mins

Cooking time: 25 mins

Servings: 4

Ingredients:

- 4 boneless, skinless chicken breasts
- 2 cups (60g) fresh spinach, chopped
- 1/2 cup (75g) feta cheese, crumbled
- 1/4 cup (37g) sun-dried tomatoes, chopped
- 2 pieces garlic, crushed
- 1 tsp (5 ml) dried oregano
- Salt and pepper as required
- Olive oil for brushing

Directions:

1. Warm up the oven to 375 deg.F.(190 deg.C.)
2. Inside your container, blend together chopped spinach, feta cheese, sun-dried tomatoes, crushed garlic, dried oregano, salt, and pepper.

3. Cut a pocket into each chicken breast.

4. Stuff each chicken breast with your spinach and feta solution.

5. Brush the outside of the chicken breasts with olive oil then flavour using salt and pepper.

6. Put filled chicken breasts in your baking dish then bake for 20-25 mins or 'til the chicken is fully cooked.

7. Present hot.

Per serving: 300 kcal; Fat: 15g; Carbs: 4g; Protein: 35g; Fiber: 2g; Sugar: 2g; Sodium: 400mg; Glycemic Index: 5

---

11. Chickpea and Vegetable Curry

Preparation time: 20 mins

Cooking time: 25 mins

Servings: 6

Ingredients:

- 2 tbsps (30 ml) olive oil
- 1 onion, chopped
- 3 pieces garlic, crushed
- 1 tbsp (15 ml) fresh ginger, grated
- 2 tbsps (30 ml) curry powder
- 1 tsp (5 ml) ground cumin
- 1 tsp (5 ml) ground coriander
- 1 tin (14 oz or 400g) cubed tomatoes
- 2 tins (15 oz each or 425g each) chickpeas, drained and rinsed
- 1 cup (240 ml) coconut milk
- 2 cups mixed vegetables (such as bell peppers, carrots, peas)
- Salt and pepper as required
- Fresh cilantro for garnish
- Cooked brown rice for serving

Directions:

1. Inside your big pot, warm olive oil in a middling temp.

2. Sauté chopped onion till translucent.

3. Include crushed garlic, grated ginger, curry powder, ground cumin, and ground coriander. Cook for 2 mins.

4. Stir in cubed tomatoes, chickpeas, coconut milk, mixed vegetables, salt, and pepper.

5. Simmer for 20-25 mins or 'til the vegetables are soft.

6. You might have to make changes to the seasoning.

7. Present over cooked brown rice, garnished using fresh cilantro.

Per serving: 350 kcal; Fat: 15g; Carbs: 40g; Protein: 12g; Fiber: 10g; Sugar: 8g; Sodium: 400mg; Glycemic Index: 30

---

12. Teriyaki Tofu Stir-Fry

Preparation time: 20 mins

Cooking time: 15 mins

Servings: 4

Ingredients:

- 1 block firm tofu, pressed and cubed
- 1/2 cup (120 ml) low-sodium teriyaki sauce
- 2 tbsps (30 ml) soy sauce (low-sodium)
- 1 tbsp (15 ml) sesame oil
- 1 tbsp (8g) cornstarch
- 2 tbsps (30 ml) vegetable oil
- 1 onion, finely sliced
- 1 bell pepper, finely sliced
- 1 cup broccoli florets
- 1 carrot, julienned
- 2 pieces garlic, crushed
- 1 tsp (5 ml) ginger, grated
- Cooked brown rice for serving
- Sesame seeds for garnish

Directions:

1. Inside your container, blend together teriyaki sauce, soy sauce, sesame oil, and cornstarch. Put away.
2. Inside your big wok or griddle, warm vegetable oil in a med-high temp.
3. Include cubed tofu then cook 'til golden brown on all sides.
4. Take out tofu from the wok then put away.
5. In the same wok, sauté sliced onion, bell pepper, broccoli, julienned carrot, crushed garlic, and grated ginger till vegetables are soft-crisp.
6. Include the teriyaki sauce solution then cooked tofu back into your wok. Stir to cover everything uniformly.
7. Present over cooked brown rice then garnish with sesame seeds.

Per serving: 300 kcal; Fat: 15g; Carbs: 25g; Protein: 18g; Fiber: 6g; Sugar: 8g; Sodium: 500mg; Glycemic Index: 20

---

13.   Mediterranean Baked Fish

Preparation time: 15 mins

Cooking time: 20 mins

Servings: 4

Ingredients:

- 4 fish fillets (e.g., cod or tilapia)
- 2 tbsps (30 ml) olive oil
- 2 pieces garlic, crushed
- 1 tsp (5 ml) dried oregano
- 1 tsp (5 ml) dried thyme
- 1/2 cup (75g) cherry tomatoes, halved
- 1/4 cup (37g) Kalamata olives, sliced
- 1/4 cup (37g) feta cheese, crumbled
- Lemon wedges for serving
- Fresh parsley for garnish
- Salt and pepper as required

Directions:

1. Warm up the oven to 400 deg.F.(200 deg.C,)
2. Put fish fillets in your baking dish.
3. Inside your small container, blend together olive oil, crushed garlic, dried oregano, dried thyme, salt, and pepper.
4. sprinkle using olive oil solution over the fish fillets.
5. Scatter cherry tomatoes, Kalamata olives, and feta cheese over the fish.
6. Bake for 15-20 mins or 'til the fish is fully cooked and flakes simply.
7. Decorate with fresh parsley as a finishing touch and present with lemon wedges.

Per serving: 250 kcal; Fat: 12g; Carbs: 5g; Protein: 30g; Fiber: 2g; Sugar: 2g; Sodium: 350mg; Glycemic Index: 5

---

14.   Spaghetti Squash with Tomato Basil Sauce

Preparation time: 15 mins

Cooking time: 45 mins

Servings: 4

Ingredients:

- 1 large spaghetti squash, halved and seeds removed
- 2 tbsps (30 ml) olive oil
- 2 pieces garlic, crushed
- 1 tin (14 oz or 400g) crushed tomatoes

- 1/4 cup (15g) fresh basil, chopped
- 1 tsp (5 ml) dried oregano
- Salt and pepper as required
- Grated Parmesan cheese for garnish

Directions:

1. Warm up the oven to 375 deg.F.(190 deg.C.)
2. Brush cut sides of the spaghetti squash with olive oil and put them cut-side down on your baking sheet.
3. Roast for 40-45 mins or 'til the squash is soft and simply torn utilizing a fork.
4. Inside your saucepot, warm olive oil in a middling temp. Include crushed garlic and sauté till fragrant.
5. Pour in crushed tomatoes, include chopped basil, dried oregano, salt, and pepper. Simmer for 10 mins.
6. Use your fork to scrape cooked spaghetti squash into "noodles."
7. Present the spaghetti squash with tomato basil sauce on top.
8. Decorate with grated Parmesan cheese.

Per serving: 180 kcal; Fat: 10g; Carbs: 20g; Protein: 3g; Fiber: 5g; Sugar: 8g; Sodium: 350mg; Glycemic Index: 20

---

15.   Pesto Chicken with Roasted Vegetables

Preparation time: 20 mins

Cooking time: 25 mins

Servings: 4

Ingredients:

- 4 boneless, skinless chicken breasts
- 1/2 cup (120 ml) pesto sauce (store-bought or homemade)
- 1 lb. (450g) baby potatoes, halved
- 1 cup (150g) cherry tomatoes
- 1 zucchini, sliced
- 1 red bell pepper, sliced
- 2 tbsps (30 ml) olive oil
- Salt and pepper as required
- Fresh basil for garnish

Directions:

1. Warm up the oven to 400 deg.F.(200 deg.C.)
2. Place chicken breasts inside a container and coat them with pesto sauce.

3. Inside a distinct container, shake baby potatoes, cherry tomatoes, zucchini, and red bell pepper with olive oil, salt, and pepper.

4. Disperse the vegetables on your baking sheet.

5. Put the pesto-covered chicken breasts on the same baking sheet.

6. Roast for 25 mins or 'til the chicken is fully cooked then the vegetables are soft.

7. Decorate with fresh basil prior to presenting.

Per serving: 350 kcal; Fat: 18g; Carbs: 20g; Protein: 25g; Fiber: 4g; Sugar: 5g; Sodium: 400mg; Glycemic Index: 15

---

16. Baked Zucchini Boats with Ground Turkey

Preparation time: 20 mins

Cooking time: 25 mins

Servings: 4

Ingredients:

- 4 medium zucchinis, halved lengthwise
- 1 lb. (450g) ground turkey
- 1 onion, finely chopped
- 2 pieces garlic, crushed
- 1 cup (150g) cherry tomatoes, cubed
- 1/2 cup (120g) black beans, drained and rinsed
- 1 tsp (5 ml) ground cumin
- 1 tsp (5 ml) chili powder
- Salt and pepper as required
- 1 cup (100g) torn cheddar cheese
- Fresh cilantro for garnish

Directions:

1. Warm up the oven to 375 deg.F.(190 deg.C.)

2. Scoop out the insides of your zucchini halves to create a boat-like shape.

3. Inside your griddle, cook ground turkey till browned. Include chopped onion and crushed garlic, cooking till softened.

4. Stir in cubed cherry tomatoes, black beans, ground cumin, chili powder, salt, and pepper.

5. Fill each zucchini boat with the turkey solution.

6. Top with torn cheddar cheese.

7. Bake for 20-25 mins or 'til the zucchini is soft and the cheese is dissolved.

8. Decorate with fresh cilantro prior to presenting.

Per serving: 300 kcal; Fat: 15g; Carbs: 20g; Protein: 20g; Fiber: 5g; Sugar: 8g; Sodium: 350mg; Glycemic Index: 15

17. Lentil and Spinach Soup

Preparation time: 15 mins

Cooking time: 30 mins

Servings: 6

Ingredients:

- 1 cup (200g) dry green or brown lentils, washed and drained
- 1 onion, chopped
- 2 carrots, cubed
- 2 celery stalks, cubed
- 3 pieces garlic, crushed
- 1 tin (14 oz or 400g) cubed tomatoes
- 6 cups (1.4 liters) vegetable broth
- 1 tsp (5 ml) ground cumin
- 1 tsp (5 ml) ground coriander
- 1 tsp (5 ml) smoked paprika
- 2 cups (60g) fresh spinach, chopped
- Salt and pepper as required
- Lemon wedges for serving

Directions:

1. Inside your big pot, sauté chopped onion, carrots, and celery till softened.
2. Place crushed garlic then cook for an extra 2 mins.
3. Stir in lentils, cubed tomatoes, vegetable broth, ground cumin, ground coriander, and smoked paprika.
4. Boil, then decrease temp. then simmer for 25-30 mins or 'til lentils are soft.
5. Include chopped spinach then cook 'til wilted.
6. Flavour using salt and pepper.
7. Present hot with lemon wedges.

Per serving: 250 kcal; Fat: 1g; Carbs: 45g; Protein: 15g; Fiber: 15g; Sugar: 5g; Sodium: 600mg; Glycemic Index: 25

18. Grilled Vegetable and Quinoa Bowl

Preparation time: 20 mins

Cooking time: 20 mins

Servings: 4

Ingredients:

- 1 cup (190g) quinoa, cooked
- 1 zucchini, sliced
- 1 bell pepper, sliced
- 1 eggplant, sliced
- 1 cup (150g) cherry tomatoes, halved
- 2 tbsps (30 ml) olive oil
- 1 tsp (5 ml) dried oregano
- 1 tsp (5 ml) dried thyme
- Salt and pepper as required
- 1/4 cup (30g) feta cheese, crumbled
- Fresh basil for garnish
- Balsamic glaze for drizzling

Directions:
1. Warm up the grill pan to med-high temp.
2. Inside your container, shake sliced zucchini, bell pepper, eggplant, and cherry tomatoes with olive oil, dried oregano, dried thyme, salt, and pepper.
3. Grill the vegetables 'til soft and mildly charred.
4. Organize cooked quinoa in containers and top with grilled vegetables.
5. sprinkle with crumbled feta cheese then garnish with fresh basil.
6. sprinkle with balsamic glaze prior to presenting.

Per serving: 350 kcal; Fat: 12g; Carbs: 50g; Protein: 10g; Fiber: 8g; Sugar: 5g; Sodium: 300mg; Glycemic Index: 20

---

19.   Turkey and Vegetable Skillet

Preparation time: 15 mins

Cooking time: 20 mins

Servings: 4

Ingredients:
- 1 lb. (450g) ground turkey
- 1 onion, chopped
- 2 bell peppers, sliced
- 1 zucchini, sliced
- 2 pieces garlic, crushed
- 1 tin (14 oz or 400g) cubed tomatoes
- 1 tsp (5 ml) ground cumin
- 1 tsp (5 ml) chili powder
- Salt and pepper as required

- Fresh cilantro for garnish
- Cooked brown rice for serving

Directions:

1. Inside your big griddle, brown ground turkey in a med-high temp.
2. Include chopped onion and crushed garlic, cooking till softened.
3. Stir in sliced bell peppers, zucchini, cubed tomatoes, ground cumin, chili powder, salt, and pepper.
4. Simmer for 15-20 mins or 'til vegetables are soft.
5. You might have to make changes to the seasoning.
6. Present over cooked brown rice then garnish with fresh cilantro.

Per serving: 300 kcal; Fat: 15g; Carbs: 20g; Protein: 25g; Fiber: 5g; Sugar: 8g; Sodium: 450mg; Glycemic Index: 20

---

20. Broiled Lemon Garlic Tilapia

Preparation time: 10 mins

Cooking time: 10 mins

Servings: 4

Ingredients:

- 4 tilapia fillets
- 2 tbsp (30 ml) olive oil
- Zest and juice of 1 lemon
- 3 pieces garlic, crushed
- 1 tsp (5 ml) dried oregano
- Salt and pepper as required
- Fresh parsley for garnish
- Lemon wedges for serving

Directions:

1. Warm up the broiler in your oven.
2. Inside your container, blend together olive oil, lemon zest, lemon juice, crushed garlic, dried oregano, salt, and pepper.
3. Place tilapia fillets on your baking sheet covered with foil.
4. Brush the fillets with the lemon-garlic solution.
5. Broil for 5-7 mins on each side or 'til the tilapia is fully cooked and flakes simply.
6. Decorate with fresh parsley as a finishing touch and present with lemon wedges.

Per serving: 180 kcal; Fat: 8g; Carbs: 1g; Protein: 25g; Fiber: 0g; Sugar: 0g; Sodium: 250mg; Glycemic Index: 0

CHAPTER 5: Snack Recipes

1.   Veggie Sticks with Hummus

Preparation time: 10 mins

Cooking time: 0 mins

Servings: 4

Ingredients:

- 2 cucumbers, cut into sticks
- 2 bell peppers (varied colors), sliced
- 1 cup (150g) cherry tomatoes
- 1 cup (240g) hummus (store-bought or homemade)

Directions:

1. Organize carrot sticks, cucumber sticks, bell pepper slices, and cherry tomatoes on a serving platter.
2. Present with a bowl of hummus for soaking.

Per serving: 150 kcal; Fat: 8g; Carbs: 18g; Protein: 6g; Fiber: 6g; Sugar: 7g; Sodium: 300mg; Glycemic Index: 15

---

2.   Almonds and Walnuts Mix

Preparation time: 5 mins

Cooking time: 0 mins

Servings: 4

Ingredients:

- 1/2 cup (70g) almonds, raw
- 1/2 cup (60g) walnuts, raw

Directions:

1. Inside your container, blend together raw almonds and walnuts.
2. Portion into small snack-sized bags for easy grab-and-go.

Per serving: 200 kcal; Fat: 18g; Carbs: 5g; Protein: 6g; Fiber: 3g; Sugar: 1g; Sodium: 0mg; Glycemic Index: 0

---

3.   Hard-Boiled Eggs with Cherry Tomatoes

Preparation time: 15 mins

Cooking time: 0 mins

Servings: 4

Ingredients:

- 4 hard-boiled eggs
- 1 cup (150g) cherry tomatoes
- Salt and pepper as required

Directions:
1. Peel the hard-boiled eggs and cut them in half.
2. Organize the egg halves and cherry tomatoes on a plate.
3. sprinkle using salt and pepper as required.

Per serving: 140 kcal; Fat: 10g; Carbs: 6g; Protein: 8g; Fiber: 2g; Sugar: 3g; Sodium: 120mg; Glycemic Index: 0

---

4. Apple Slices with Peanut Butter

Preparation time: 5 mins

Cooking time: 0 mins

Servings: 2

Ingredients:
- 2 apples, sliced
- 4 tbsp (60 ml) natural peanut butter

Directions:
1. Slice the apples into thin wedges.
2. Present with individual portions of natural peanut butter for soaking.

Per serving: 250 kcal; Fat: 16g; Carbs: 25g; Protein: 5g; Fiber: 6g; Sugar: 18g; Sodium: 80mg; Glycemic Index: 10

---

5. Roasted Chickpeas with Spices

Preparation time: 10 mins

Cooking time: 30 mins

Servings: 4

Ingredients:
- 2 tins (15 oz each or 425g each) chickpeas, drained and rinsed
- 2 tbsp (30 ml) olive oil
- 1 tsp (5 ml) ground cumin
- 1 tsp (5 ml) smoked paprika
- 1/2 tsp (2.5 ml) cayenne pepper (adjust as required)
- Salt as required

Directions:
1. Warm up the oven to 400 deg.F.(200 deg.C.)

2. Pat chickpeas dry using a paper towel to take out extra moisture.

3. Inside your container, shake chickpeas with olive oil, ground cumin, smoked paprika, cayenne pepper, and salt.

4. Disperse the chickpeas on your baking sheet in a single layer.

5. Roast for 25-30 mins or 'til chickpeas are crispy, shaking the pan halfway through for even cooking.

6. Allow to cool prior to presenting.

Per serving: 180 kcal; Fat: 8g; Carbs: 22g; Protein: 7g; Fiber: 6g; Sugar: 4g; Sodium: 300mg; Glycemic Index: 25

---

6. Edamame with Sea Salt

Preparation time: 5 mins

Cooking time: 5 mins

Servings: 4

Ingredients:

- 2 cups (300g) frozen edamame, thawed
- Sea salt as required

Directions:

1. Boil or steam edamame using the package guidelines.

2. sprinkle with sea salt while still warm.

3. Present inside a container.

Per serving: 120 kcal; Fat: 4g; Carbs: 10g; Protein: 12g; Fiber: 6g; Sugar: 2g; Sodium: 5mg; Glycemic Index: 10

---

7. Avocado Salsa with Whole Wheat Crackers

Preparation time: 10 mins

Cooking time: 0 mins

Servings: 2

Ingredients:

- 2 avocados, cubed
- 1 cup (150g) cherry tomatoes, cubed
- 1/4 cup (40g) red onion, finely chopped
- 1/4 cup (15g) cilantro, chopped
- 1 jalapeño, seeds removed and finely chopped
- Juice of 1 lime
- Salt and pepper as required
- Whole wheat crackers for serving

Directions:

1. Inside your container, blend cubed avocados, cherry tomatoes, red onion, cilantro, and jalapeño.
2. sprinkle lime juice over the solution and carefully shake.
3. Flavour using salt and pepper as required.
4. Present with whole wheat crackers.

Per serving: 300 kcal; Fat: 24g; Carbs: 20g; Protein: 5g; Fiber: 12g; Sugar: 3g; Sodium: 150mg; Glycemic Index: 15

---

8.   Trail Mix with Nuts and Seeds

Preparation time: 5 mins

Cooking time: 0 mins

Servings: 4

Ingredients:

- 1/2 cup (70g) almonds, raw
- 1/2 cup (60g) walnuts, raw
- 1/4 cup (30g) pumpkin seeds
- 1/4 cup (30g) sunflower seeds
- 1/4 cup (30g) dried cranberries (unsweetened)

Directions:

1. Inside your container, blend together raw almonds, walnuts, pumpkin seeds, sunflower seeds, and dried cranberries.
2. Portion into small snack-sized bags for easy grab-and-go.

Per serving: 250 kcal; Fat: 20g; Carbs: 15g; Protein: 8g; Fiber: 4g; Sugar: 6g; Sodium: 5mg; Glycemic Index: 10

---

9.   Cherry Almond Energy Bites

Preparation time: 15 mins

Cooking time: 0 mins

Servings: 12

Ingredients:

- 1 cup (90g) rolled oats
- 1/2 cup (120 ml) almond butter
- 1/3 cup (80 ml) honey or maple syrup
- 1/2 cup (75g) dried cherries, chopped
- 1/4 cup (30g) almonds, finely chopped
- 1 tsp (5 ml) vanilla extract

- Pinch of salt

Directions:

1. Inside your container, blend together rolled oats, vanilla extract, almond butter, honey (or maple syrup), dried cherries, chopped almonds, and a tweak of salt.
2. Put in the fridge the solution for 15-30 mins as a means of making it more manageable.
3. Roll the solution into bite-sized balls.
4. Store in your airtight container in the fridge.

Per serving: 150 kcal; Fat: 8g; Carbs: 18g; Protein: 4g; Fiber: 2g; Sugar: 9g; Sodium: 10mg; Glycemic Index: 20

---

10. Cucumber and Tomato Salad

Preparation time: 10 mins

Cooking time: 0 mins

Servings: 4

Ingredients:

- 2 cucumbers, sliced
- 2 cups (300g) cherry tomatoes, halved
- 1/4 cup (40g) red onion, finely sliced
- 1/4 cup (30g) feta cheese, crumbled
- 2 tbsps (30 ml) olive oil
- 1 tbsp (15 ml) balsamic vinegar
- 1 tsp (5 ml) dried oregano
- Salt and pepper as required
- Fresh basil for garnish

Directions:

1. Inside your container, blend sliced cucumbers, cherry tomatoes, red onion, and crumbled feta cheese.
2. Inside your small container, whisk together olive oil, balsamic vinegar, dried oregano, salt, and pepper.
3. sprinkle using dressing over the salad then shake carefully.
4. Decorate with fresh basil prior to presenting.

Per serving: 120 kcal; Fat: 9g; Carbs: 9g; Protein: 3g; Fiber: 2g; Sugar: 5g; Sodium: 150mg; Glycemic Index: 10

---

11. Mini Caprese Skewers

Preparation time: 15 mins

Cooking time: 0 mins

Servings: 4

Ingredients:

- 16 cherry tomatoes
- 16 small fresh mozzarella balls
- 16 small basil leaves
- Balsamic glaze for drizzling

Directions:

1. Attach a cherry tomato, a fresh mozzarella ball, and a basil leaf to little skewers and string them together.
2. Organize the skewers on a serving platter.
3. sprinkle with balsamic glaze prior to presenting.

Per serving: 150 kcal; Fat: 10g; Carbs: 5g; Protein: 8g; Fiber: 1g; Sugar: 2g; Sodium: 150mg; Glycemic Index: 5

12. Baked Kale Chips

Preparation time: 10 mins

Cooking time: 15 mins

Servings: 2

Ingredients:

- 1 bunch kale, stems removed and torn into bite-sized pieces
- 1 tbsp (15 ml) olive oil
- 1 tsp (5 ml) garlic powder
- 1/2 tsp (2.5 ml) smoked paprika
- Salt as required

Directions:

1. Warm up the oven to 350 deg.F.(180 deg.C.)
2. Inside your container, shake kale pieces with olive oil, garlic powder, smoked paprika, and salt.
3. Disperse the kale on your baking sheet in a single layer.
4. Bake for 10-15 mins or 'til the edges are crispy but not burnt.
5. Allow to cool prior to presenting.

Per serving: 100 kcal; Fat: 7g; Carbs: 8g; Protein: 3g; Fiber: 2g; Sugar: 0g; Sodium: 150mg; Glycemic Index: 5

13. Sliced Bell Peppers with Guacamole

Preparation time: 10 mins

Cooking time: 0 mins

Servings: 4

Ingredients:

- 2 bell peppers (assorted colors), sliced
- 2 avocados, mashed
- 1 tomato, cubed
- 1/4 cup (40g) red onion, finely chopped
- 1 piece garlic, crushed
- Juice of 1 lime
- Salt and pepper as required
- Fresh cilantro for garnish

Directions:

1. Organize sliced bell peppers on a serving platter.
2. Inside your container, blend together mashed avocados, cubed tomato, red onion, crushed garlic, lime juice, salt, and pepper.
3. Spoon guacamole onto each bell pepper slice.
4. Decorate with fresh cilantro prior to presenting.

Per serving: 150 kcal; Fat: 12g; Carbs: 12g; Protein: 2g; Fiber: 7g; Sugar: 2g; Sodium: 10mg; Glycemic Index: 10

---

14. Greek Salad Skewers

Preparation time: 15 mins

Cooking time: 0 mins

Servings: 4

Ingredients:

- 1 cup (150g) cherry tomatoes
- 1 cucumber, sliced
- 1 cup (150g) Kalamata olives
- 1 cup (150g) feta cheese, cubed
- 1/4 cup (40g) red onion, finely sliced
- Olive oil for drizzling
- Fresh oregano for garnish

Directions:

1. Thread cherry tomatoes, cucumber slices, Kalamata olives, feta cheese cubes, and red onion onto small skewers.

2. Organize the skewers on a serving platter.
3. sprinkle with olive oil then garnish with fresh oregano.

Per serving: 200 kcal; Fat: 15g; Carbs: 10g; Protein: 8g; Fiber: 3g; Sugar: 4g; Sodium: 500mg; Glycemic Index: 15

---

15. Quinoa and Black Bean Salad Cups

Preparation time: 20 mins

Cooking time: 15 mins

Servings: 4

Ingredients:

- 1 cup (190g) quinoa, cooked
- 1 tin (15 oz or 425g) black beans, drained and rinsed
- 1 cup (150g) corn kernels (fresh or frozen)
- 1 red bell pepper, cubed
- 1/4 cup (40g) red onion, finely chopped
- 1/4 cup (15g) fresh cilantro, chopped
- Juice of 1 lime
- 2 tbsps (30 ml) olive oil
- Salt and pepper as required
- Butter lettuce leaves for serving

Directions:

1. Inside your container, blend cooked quinoa, black beans, corn kernels, cubed red bell pepper, red onion, and chopped cilantro.
2. Inside your small container, whisk together lime juice, olive oil, salt, and pepper. Pour over the quinoa solution then shake to blend.
3. Spoon the quinoa and black bean salad into butter lettuce leaves to create cups.
4. Present chilled.

Per serving: 250 kcal; Fat: 8g; Carbs: 38g; Protein: 9g; Fiber: 8g; Sugar: 4g; Sodium: 300mg; Glycemic Index: 20

---

16. Smoked Salmon Cucumber Bites

Preparation time: 10 mins

Cooking time: 0 mins

Servings: 4

Ingredients:

- 1 English cucumber, sliced

- 4 oz (115g) smoked salmon, cut into small pieces
- 1/4 cup (60g) cream cheese
- 1 tbsp (5g) fresh dill, chopped
- Lemon wedges for serving

Directions:

1. Organize cucumber slices on a serving platter.
2. Disperse a small amount of cream cheese on each cucumber slice.
3. Top with pieces of smoked salmon.
4. Decorate with fresh dill and present with lemon wedges.

Per serving: 150 kcal; Fat: 10g; Carbs: 5g; Protein: 10g; Fiber: 1g; Sugar: 2g; Sodium: 400mg; Glycemic Index: 0

---

17. Celery Sticks with Cream Cheese

Preparation time: 10 mins

Cooking time: 0 mins

Servings: 2

Ingredients:

- 4 celery stalks, cut into sticks
- 1/2 cup (120g) cream cheese, softened
- 1 tbsp (3g) chives, chopped (optional)
- Black pepper as required

Directions:

1. Disperse a generous amount of your softened cream cheese on each celery stick.
2. sprinkle with chopped chives and black pepper.
3. Present chilled.

Per serving: 120 kcal; Fat: 10g; Carbs: 4g; Protein: 2g; Fiber: 2g; Sugar: 2g; Sodium: 100mg; Glycemic Index: 0

---

18. Roasted Pumpkin Seeds

Preparation time: 5 mins

Cooking time: 15 mins

Servings: 4

Ingredients:

- 1 cup (130g) pumpkin seeds, raw and unsalted
- 1 tbsp (15 ml) olive oil
- 1/2 tsp (2.5 ml) garlic powder

- 1/2 tsp (2.5 ml) paprika
- Salt as required

Directions:

1. Warm up the oven to 300 deg.F.(160 deg.C.)
2. Inside your container, shake pumpkin seeds with olive oil, garlic powder, paprika, and salt.
3. Disperse seeds on your baking sheet in a single layer.
4. Roast for 15 mins or 'til golden and crispy.
5. Allow to cool prior to presenting.

Per serving: 180 kcal; Fat: 15g; Carbs: 4g; Protein: 8g; Fiber: 2g; Sugar: 0g; Sodium: 50mg; Glycemic Index: 0

---

19. Whole Grain Rice Cake with Cottage Cheese

Preparation time: 5 mins

Cooking time: 0 mins

Servings: 2

Ingredients:

- 2 whole grain rice cakes
- 1/2 cup (120g) low-fat cottage cheese
- 1/2 cup (75g) cherry tomatoes, halved
- 1 tbsp (3g) chives, chopped
- Black pepper as required

Directions:

1. Disperse a layer of your cottage cheese on each whole grain rice cake.
2. Top with divided cherry tomatoes.
3. sprinkle with chopped chives and black pepper.
4. Present instantly.

Per serving: 150 kcal; Fat: 3g; Carbs: 25g; Protein: 7g; Fiber: 3g; Sugar: 3g; Sodium: 200mg; Glycemic Index: 40

---

20. Eggplant Lasagna

Preparation time: 20 mins

Cooking time: 40 mins

Servings: 4

Ingredients:

- 1 large eggplant, finely sliced lengthwise
- 1 lb. (450g) lean ground beef
- 1 onion, chopped

- 2 pieces garlic, crushed
- 1 tin (14 oz or 400g) crushed tomatoes
- 1 tsp (5 ml) dried oregano
- 1 tsp (5 ml) dried basil
- Salt and pepper as required
- 1 cup (240g) part-skim ricotta cheese
- 1 cup (100g) torn mozzarella cheese
- Fresh basil for garnish

Directions:

1. Warm up the oven to 375 deg.F.(190 deg.C.)
2. Inside your griddle, brown the ground beef in a middling temp. Include chopped onion and crushed garlic, cooking till softened.
3. Stir in crushed tomatoes, dried oregano, dried basil, salt, and pepper. Simmer for 10 mins.
4. Inside an oiled baking dish, layer sliced eggplant, ricotta cheese, meat sauce, and torn mozzarella cheese. Repeat 'til all components are used, finishing with a layer of mozzarella on top.
5. Bake for 30-40 mins or 'til the cheese is dissolved and bubbly.
6. Decorate with fresh basil prior to presenting.

Per serving: 350 kcal; Fat: 15g; Carbs: 20g; Protein: 30g; Fiber: 8g; Sugar: 10g; Sodium: 500mg; Glycemic Index: 30

CHAPTER 6: Dessert Recipes

1.   Baked Apples with Cinnamon

Preparation time: 10 mins

Cooking time: 25 mins

Servings: 2

Ingredients:

- 2 apples, cored and halved
- 1 tbsp (15 ml) melted coconut oil
- 1 tsp (5 ml) ground cinnamon
- 1 tbsp (8g) chopped nuts (optional)
- 1 tbsp (15 ml) honey or maple syrup (optional)

Directions:

1. Warm up the oven to 375 deg.F.(190 deg.C.)
2. Put apple halves on your baking sheet.
3. Brush dissolved coconut oil over the apples.
4. sprinkle ground cinnamon uniformly over each apple half.
5. Bake for 25 mins or 'til apples are soft.
6. Optional: sprinkle chopped nuts and sprinkle honey or maple syrup prior to presenting.

Per serving: 150 kcal; Fat: 5g; Carbs: 30g; Protein: 1g; Fiber: 5g; Sugar: 20g; Sodium: 0mg; Glycemic Index: 35

---

2.   Dark Chocolate-Dipped Strawberries

Preparation time: 15 mins

Cooking time: 0 mins

Servings: 4

Ingredients:

- 1 cup (175g) dark chocolate chips
- 1 tbsp (15 ml) coconut oil
- 16 fresh strawberries, washed and dried

Directions:

1. Inside a microwave-safe container, dissolve dark chocolate chips and coconut oil in 30-second intervals, mixing till smooth.
2. Dip each strawberry into your dissolved chocolate, covering half of the strawberry.
3. Place dipped strawberries on a parchment paper-covered tray.

4. Chill in the fridge for 30 mins or 'til the chocolate hardens.

Per serving: 180 kcal; Fat: 12g; Carbs: 20g; Protein: 2g; Fiber: 4g; Sugar: 12g; Sodium: 0mg; Glycemic Index: 40

---

3.   Coconut Flour Banana Bread

Preparation time: 15 mins

Cooking time: 40 mins

Servings: 8

Ingredients:

- 3 ripe bananas, mashed
- 3 eggs
- 1/4 cup (60 ml) coconut oil, melted
- 1/4 cup (60 ml) honey or maple syrup
- 1 tsp (5 ml) vanilla extract
- 1/2 cup (60g) coconut flour
- 1/2 tsp (2.5 ml) baking soda
- 1/4 tsp (1.25 ml) salt
- 1/2 cup (60g) chopped walnuts (optional)

Directions:

1. Warm up the oven to 350 deg.F.(180 deg.C.) Grease a loaf pan.
2. Inside your container, whisk together honey or maple syrup, mashed bananas, eggs, dissolved coconut oil, and vanilla extract.
3. Inside a different bowl, blend coconut flour, baking soda, and salt.
4. Put the dry components into your wet components and stir till well blended.
5. Fold in chopped walnuts if anticipated.
6. Pour the batter into your oiled loaf pan and smooth the top.
7. Bake for 40 mins or 'til a toothpick immersed into your center comes out clean.
8. Allow to cool prior to slicing.

Per serving: 220 kcal; Fat: 12g; Carbs: 26g; Protein: 4g; Fiber: 4g; Sugar: 16g; Sodium: 180mg; Glycemic Index: 30

---

4.   Almond Flour Blueberry Muffins

Preparation time: 15 mins

Cooking time: 25 mins

Servings: 6

Ingredients:

- 2 cups (200g) almond flour
- 1/4 cup (30g) coconut flour
- 1/2 tsp (2.5 ml) baking soda
- 1/4 tsp (1.25 ml) salt
- 3 eggs
- 1/4 cup (60 ml) coconut oil, melted
- 1/4 cup (60 ml) honey or maple syrup
- 1 tsp (5 ml) vanilla extract
- 1 cup (150g) fresh blueberries

Directions:

1. Warm up the oven to 350 deg.F.(180 deg.C.) Line a muffin tin with paper liners.
2. Inside your container, whisk together almond flour, coconut flour, baking soda, and salt.
3. Inside a distinct container, honey or maple syrup, dissolved coconut oil, beat eggs, and vanilla extract.
4. Put the wet components into your dry components and mix till well blended.
5. Fold in fresh blueberries.
6. Spoon the batter into your muffin cups, filling each about two-thirds full.
7. Bake for 25 mins or 'til a toothpick immersed into your center comes out clean.
8. Allow to cool prior to presenting.

Per serving: 280 kcal; Fat: 22g; Carbs: 16g; Protein: 8g; Fiber: 4g; Sugar: 9g; Sodium: 180mg; Glycemic Index: 25

---

5.   Chocolate Avocado Mousse

Preparation time: 10 mins

Cooking time: 0 mins

Servings: 4

Ingredients:

- 2 ripe avocados, peeled and pitted
- 1/2 cup (50g) unsweetened cocoa powder
- 1/2 cup (120 ml) almond milk
- 1/4 cup (60 ml) honey or maple syrup
- 1 tsp (5 ml) vanilla extract
- Pinch of salt
- Fresh berries for garnish (optional)

Directions:

1. Inside a mixer, blend avocados, cocoa powder, almond milk, honey or maple syrup, vanilla extract, and a tweak of salt.

2. Blend till smooth and creamy.
3. Chill the mousse in your fridge for almost 2 hrs.
4. Present topped with fresh berries if anticipated.

Per serving: 200 kcal; Fat: 15g; Carbs: 20g; Protein: 4g; Fiber: 8g; Sugar: 8g; Sodium: 50mg; Glycemic Index: 20

---

6. Pumpkin Spice Chia Seed Pudding

Preparation time: 10 mins

Cooking time: 0 mins

Servings: 2

Ingredients:

- 1/4 cup (40g) chia seeds
- 1 cup (240 ml) unsweetened almond milk
- 1/2 cup (120g) tinned pumpkin puree
- 2 tbsps (30 ml) maple syrup
- 1/2 tsp (2.5 ml) pumpkin spice
- 1/2 tsp (2.5 ml) vanilla extract
- Pecans or walnuts for garnish (optional)

Directions:

1. Inside your container, whisk together chia seeds, almond milk, pumpkin puree, maple syrup, pumpkin spice, and vanilla extract.
2. Let the solution sit for 10 mins, then whisk again to prevent clumping.
3. Cover then put in the fridge for almost 4 hrs or overnight.
4. Present chilled, garnished using nuts if anticipated.

Per serving: 80 kcal; Fat: 8g; Carbs: 25g; Protein: 5g; Fiber: 12g; Sugar: 10g; Sodium: 80mg; Glycemic Index: 20

---

7. Mixed Berry Sorbet

Preparation time: 10 mins

Cooking time: 0 mins

Servings: 4

Ingredients:

- 2 cups (300g) mixed berries (strawberries, blueberries, raspberries)
- 1/4 cup (60 ml) honey or maple syrup
- 1 tbsp (15 ml) fresh lemon juice
- 1/2 cup (120 ml) water

Directions:

1. Inside a mixer, blend mixed berries, honey or maple syrup, lemon juice, and water.
2. Blend till smooth.
3. Pour solution into your shallow dish and freeze for 4 hrs, mixing every hr to break up ice crystals.
4. Scoop and present as a refreshing sorbet.

Per serving: 80 kcal; Fat: 0g; Carbs: 20g; Protein: 1g; Fiber: 4g; Sugar: 15g; Sodium: 0mg; Glycemic Index: 30

8.　Vanilla Bean Panna Cotta

Preparation time: 15 mins

Cooking time: 0 mins

Servings: 4

Ingredients:

- 1 cup (240 ml) coconut milk
- 1 cup (240 ml) almond milk
- 1/4 cup (60 ml) honey or maple syrup
- 1 tsp (5 ml) vanilla extract
- 2 tsps (6g) unflavored gelatin powder
- Fresh mint for garnish (optional)

Directions:

1. Inside your saucepot, heat almond milk, honey or maple syrup, coconut milk, and vanilla extract in a middling temp. 'til warm but not boiling.
2. Inside your small container, sprinkle gelatin over 2 tbsps of water and let it bloom for a couple of mins.
3. Include the bloomed gelatin to your milk solution, mixing till completely dissolved.
4. Take out from temp. and allow it to relax for 5 mins.
5. Pour solution into serving glasses and put in the fridge for almost 4 hrs or 'til set.
6. Decorate with fresh mint prior to presenting.

Per serving: 150 kcal; Fat: 9g; Carbs: 15g; Protein: 3g; Fiber: 0g; Sugar: 12g; Sodium: 30mg; Glycemic Index: 25

9.　Lemon Poppy Seed Almond Cake

Preparation time: 15 mins

Cooking time: 30 mins

Servings: 8

Ingredients:

- 1 cup (100g) almond flour

- 1/4 cup (30g) coconut flour
- 1/2 tsp (2.5 ml) baking soda
- 1/4 tsp (1.25 ml) salt
- 3 eggs
- 1/4 cup (60 ml) coconut oil, melted
- 1/4 cup (60 ml) honey or maple syrup
- Zest of 1 lemon
- 2 tbsps (30 ml) lemon juice
- 1 tbsp (10g) poppy seeds

Directions:

1. Warm up the oven to 350 deg.F.(180 deg.C.) Grease a cake pan.
2. Inside your container, whisk together almond flour, coconut flour, baking soda, and salt.
3. Inside a distinct container, beat eggs, dissolved coconut oil, honey or maple syrup, lemon zest, and lemon juice.
4. Blend wet & dry components, then wrap in poppy seeds.
5. Pour the batter into your oiled cake pan then bake for 30 mins or 'til a toothpick immersed into your center comes out clean.
6. Allow the cake to cool prior to slicing.

Per serving: 200 kcal; Fat: 16g; Carbs: 11g; Protein: 6g; Fiber: 3g; Sugar: 7g; Sodium: 150mg; Glycemic Index: 15

10.　Ricotta and Berry Parfait

Preparation time: 10 mins

Cooking time: 0 mins

Servings: 2

Ingredients:

- 1 cup (240g) low-fat ricotta cheese
- 1 tbsp (15 ml) honey or maple syrup
- 1/2 tsp (2.5 ml) vanilla extract
- 1 cup (150g) mixed berries (strawberries, blueberries, raspberries)
- Mint leaves for garnish (optional)

Directions:

1. Inside your container, blend together ricotta cheese, honey or maple syrup, and vanilla extract.
2. In serving glasses, layer the ricotta solution with mixed berries.
3. Repeat layers then finish using a layer of berries on top.
4. Decorate with mint leaves if anticipated.

Per serving: 220 kcal; Fat: 10g; Carbs: 20g; Protein: 12g; Fiber: 4g; Sugar: 12g; Sodium: 100mg; Glycemic Index: 20

---

11.   Pistachio and Cranberry Biscotti

Preparation time: 15 mins

Cooking time: 30 mins

Servings: 12

Ingredients:

- 1 cup (100g) almond flour
- 1/4 cup (30g) coconut flour
- 1/4 cup (30g) pistachios, chopped
- 1/4 cup (30g) dried cranberries, chopped
- 1/4 cup (60 ml) honey or maple syrup
- 1 egg
- 1/2 tsp (2.5 ml) vanilla extract
- 1/4 tsp (1.25 ml) baking soda
- Pinch of salt

Directions:

1. Warm up the oven to 325 deg.F.(179 deg.C.) Cover a baking surface with parchment paper and set it aside.
2. Inside your container, blend almond flour, coconut flour, chopped pistachios, baking soda, chopped cranberries, honey or maple syrup, egg, vanilla extract, and a tweak of salt.
3. Form the dough into a log shape on the prepared baking sheet.
4. Bake for 25-30 mins or 'til the edges are golden.
5. Let the log to cool for 10 mins, then slice into biscotti shapes.
6. Put the slices back on the baking sheet then bake for an extra 10 mins or 'til crisp.
7. Cool completely prior to presenting.

Per serving: 120 kcal; Fat: 8g; Carbs: 11g; Protein: 4g; Fiber: 2g; Sugar: 7g; Sodium: 50mg; Glycemic Index: 15

---

12.   Greek Yogurt and Honey Frozen Drops

Preparation time: 5 mins

Cooking time: 0 mins

Servings: 4

Ingredients:

- 1 cup (240g) Greek yogurt

- 2 tbsps (30 ml) honey
- 1/2 tsp (2.5 ml) vanilla extract

Directions:

1. Inside your container, blend together Greek yogurt, honey, and vanilla extract.
2. Cover a baking surface with parchment paper and set it aside.
3. Spoon small drops of the yogurt solution into your parchment paper.
4. Freeze for almost 2 hrs or 'til solid.
5. Present as frozen yogurt drops.

Per serving: 80 kcal; Fat: 2g; Carbs: 12g; Protein: 4g; Fiber: 0g; Sugar: 11g; Sodium: 20mg; Glycemic Index: 10

---

13.   Avocado Lime Cheesecake Bites

Preparation time: 20 mins

Cooking time: 0 mins

Servings: 12

Ingredients:

- 1 cup (140g) raw almonds
- 1 cup (150g) dates, pitted
- 1 ripe avocado
- 1/4 cup (60 ml) coconut oil, melted
- 1/4 cup (60 ml) lime juice
- Zest of 1 lime
- 1/4 cup (60 ml) honey or maple syrup
- 1 tsp (5 ml) vanilla extract
- Pinch of salt

Directions:

1. Inside a blending container, blend raw almonds till finely ground.
2. Include dates and continue to process till a sticky dough forms.
3. Press the almond-date solution into your base of a mini muffin tin to create the crust.
4. Inside a mixer, blend dissolved coconut oil, lime zest, lime juice, honey or maple syrup, ripe avocado, vanilla extract, and a tweak of salt. Blend till smooth.
5. Spoon the avocado solution into your crust in the muffin tin.
6. Chill in the fridge for almost 2 hrs prior to presenting.

Per serving: 150 kcal; Fat: 10g; Carbs: 14g; Protein: 3g; Fiber: 3g; Sugar: 9g; Sodium: 5mg; Glycemic Index: 20

---

14. Almond and Coconut Energy Balls

Preparation time: 15 mins

Cooking time: 0 mins

Servings: 10

Ingredients:

- 1 cup (140g) almonds
- 1/2 cup (40g) shredded coconut
- 1/4 cup (60g) almond butter
- 2 tbsps (30 ml) honey or maple syrup
- 1/2 tsp (2.5 ml) vanilla extract
- Pinch of salt

Directions:

1. Inside a blending container, pulse almonds and torn coconut till finely ground.
2. Include almond butter, honey or maple syrup, vanilla extract, and a tweak of salt. Blend till the solution comes together.
3. Roll the solution into small energy balls.
4. Chill in your fridge for almost 30 mins prior to presenting.

Per serving: 150 kcal; Fat: 12g; Carbs: 8g; Protein: 5g; Fiber: 3g; Sugar: 4g; Sodium: 5mg; Glycemic Index: 15

---

15. Baked Pears with Cinnamon and Walnuts

Preparation time: 10 mins

Cooking time: 20 mins

Servings: 4

Ingredients:

- 2 pears, halved and cored
- 1 tbsp (15 ml) coconut oil, melted
- 1 tsp (5 ml) ground cinnamon
- 1/4 cup (30g) chopped walnuts
- 2 tbsps (30 ml) honey or maple syrup

Directions:

1. Warm up the oven to 375 deg.F.(190 deg.C.) Put pear halves in your baking dish.
2. Inside your small container, mix dissolved coconut oil and ground cinnamon.
3. Brush the cinnamon solution over each pear half.
4. sprinkle chopped walnuts over the pears and sprinkle with honey or maple syrup.
5. Bake for 20 mins or 'til the pears are soft.
6. Present warm.

Per serving: 150 kcal; Fat: 9g; Carbs: 18g; Protein: 2g; Fiber: 4g; Sugar: 11g; Sodium: 0mg; Glycemic Index: 20

---

16.   Raspberry Almond Crumble Bars

Preparation time: 15 mins

Cooking time: 30 mins

Servings: 9

Ingredients:

- 1 cup (100g) almond flour
- 1/4 cup (30g) coconut flour
- 1/4 cup (60 ml) coconut oil, melted
- 2 tbsps (30 ml) honey or maple syrup
- 1 tsp (5 ml) vanilla extract
- Pinch of salt
- 1 cup (150g) fresh or frozen raspberries

Directions:

1. Warm up the oven to 350 deg.F.(180 deg.C.) Line a baking pan using parchment paper.
2. Inside your container, blend almond flour, coconut flour, dissolved coconut oil, honey or maple syrup, vanilla extract, and a tweak of salt. Mix till crumbly.
3. Press two-thirds of the solution into the bottom of your prepared pan to create the crust.
4. Scatter raspberries uniformly over the crust.
5. sprinkle the remaining crumble solution over the raspberries.
6. Bake for 30 mins or 'til the top is golden brown.
7. Allow to cool prior to cutting into bars.

Per serving: 180 kcal; Fat: 14g; Carbs: 12g; Protein: 4g; Fiber: 3g; Sugar: 7g; Sodium: 40mg; Glycemic Index: 15

---

17.   Cinnamon Roasted Almonds

Preparation time: 5 mins

Cooking time: 15 mins

Servings: 4

Ingredients:

- 2 cups (280g) raw almonds
- 1 tbsp (15 ml) coconut oil, melted
- 1 tbsp (15 ml) honey or maple syrup
- 1 tsp (5 ml) ground cinnamon

- Pinch of salt

Directions:

1. Warm up the oven to 325 deg.F.(170 deg.C.) Cover a baking surface with parchment paper and set it aside.
2. Inside your container, shake raw almonds with dissolved coconut oil, honey or maple syrup, ground cinnamon, and a tweak of salt.
3. Disperse the almonds on to your prepared baking sheet in a single layer.
4. Bake for 15 mins, mixing halfway through.
5. Allow to cool prior to presenting.

Per serving: 220 kcal; Fat: 18g; Carbs: 8g; Protein: 8g; Fiber: 4g; Sugar: 2g; Sodium: 50mg; Glycemic Index: 15

---

18. Coconut and Lime Sorbet

Preparation time: 10 mins

Cooking time: 0 mins

Servings: 4

Ingredients:

- 1 tin (14 oz or 400 ml) coconut milk
- 1/4 cup (60 ml) honey or maple syrup
- Zest of 2 limes
- 1/4 cup (60 ml) lime juice

Directions:

1. Inside a mixer, blend coconut milk, honey or maple syrup, lime zest, and lime juice.
2. Blend till smooth.
3. Pour the solution into your shallow dish and freeze for 4 hrs, mixing every hr to break up ice crystals.
4. Present as a refreshing sorbet.

Per serving: 200 kcal; Fat: 18g; Carbs: 10g; Protein: 2g; Fiber: 0g; Sugar: 8g; Sodium: 20mg; Glycemic Index: 20

---

19. Strawberry and Mint Infused Water

Preparation time: 5 mins

Cooking time: 0 mins

Servings: 2

Ingredients:

- 1 cup (150g) strawberries, sliced
- 1/4 cup (10g) fresh mint leaves

- 2 cups (480 ml) water

Directions:

1. Inside a pitcher, blend sliced strawberries and fresh mint leaves.
2. Fill pitcher with 2 cups of water.
3. Put in the fridge for 2 hrs to let the flavors to infuse.
4. Present over ice.

Per serving: 10 kcal; Fat: 0g; Carbs: 3g; Protein: 0g; Fiber: 1g; Sugar: 1g; Sodium: 0mg; Glycemic Index: 5

---

20. Pecan and Date Energy Squares

Preparation time: 15 mins

Cooking time: 0 mins

Servings: 9

Ingredients:

- 1 cup (100g) pecans
- 1 cup (150g) dates, pitted
- 1/4 cup (20g) unsweetened shredded coconut
- 1 tbsp (12g) chia seeds
- 1/4 cup (60g) almond butter
- 1 tsp (5 ml) vanilla extract
- Pinch of salt

Directions:

1. Inside a blending container, blend pecans till finely ground.
2. Include dates, torn coconut, chia seeds, almond butter, vanilla extract, and a tweak of salt. Blend till the solution comes together.
3. Press the solution into a square dish to create an even layer.
4. Chill in the fridge for almost 2 hrs prior to cutting into squares.

Per serving: 150 kcal; Fat: 10g; Carbs: 15g; Protein: 3g; Fiber: 3g; Sugar: 11g; Sodium: 10mg; Glycemic Index: 20

Shopping List

Proteins:

- Smoked salmon
- Eggs
- Turkey
- Grilled chicken
- Shrimp
- Tofu
- Cod
- Ground turkey
- Tilapia

Vegetables:

- Cucumber
- Bell peppers
- Zucchini
- Spinach
- Mushrooms
- Asparagus
- Broccoli
- Radish
- Eggplant
- Cherry tomatoes
- Lettuce
- Avocado
- Onion

Fruits:

- Banana
- Berries (blueberries, strawberries, raspberries)
- Apple
- Lemon
- Lime

Whole Grains:

- Quinoa
- Oat bran
- Whole grain toast
- Whole wheat pasta
- Spaghetti squash
- Brown rice

Legumes:

- Black beans
- Chickpeas
- Lentils

Dairy and Alternatives:

- Cottage cheese
- Feta cheese
- Parmesan cheese
- Greek yogurt

Nuts and Seeds:

- Almonds
- Walnuts
- Pistachios
- Chia seeds
- Pumpkin seeds
- Coconut flour

Healthy Fats:

- Olive oil
- Avocado oil
- Coconut oil

Herbs and Spices:

- Cinnamon
- Basil
- Dill
- Garlic
- Paprika
- Cumin
- Turmeric

Condiments:

- Hummus
- Pesto
- Salsa
- Balsamic glaze
- Teriyaki sauce

Beverages:

- Green tea
- Infused water

Sweeteners:

- Honey

- Dark chocolate

Other Snacks:

- Edamame
- Whole grain rice cakes

- Whole wheat crackers

Miscellaneous:

- Sea salt
- Ground black pepper

30 Day Meal Plan

Day	Breakfast	Lunch	Dinner	Dessert
1	Veggie Omelet Muffins	Quinoa and Black Bean Stuffed Peppers	Grilled Salmon with Dill Sauce	Coconut Flour Banana Bread
2	Cottage Cheese Pancakes	Mediterranean Chickpea Salad	Garlic Parmesan Baked Cod	Pistachio and Cranberry Biscotti
3	Zucchini and Cheese Egg Bake	Turkey and Avocado Wrap	Chickpea and Vegetable Curry	Baked Pears with Cinnamon and Walnuts
4	Overnight Oats with Nuts and Berries	Tuna Salad Lettuce Wraps	Quinoa-Stuffed Bell Peppers	Vanilla Bean Panna Cotta
5	Almond Flour Pancakes	Cauliflower Rice Stir-Fry with Tofu	Lemon Garlic Shrimp Skewers	Dark Chocolate-Dipped Strawberries
6	Banana Walnut Muffins	Grilled Veggie and Hummus Wrap	Greek Quinoa Salad	Almond and Coconut Energy Balls
7	Berry and Spinach Smoothie Bowl	Caprese Salad with Balsamic Glaze	Zucchini Noodles with Pesto and Cherry Tomatoes	Raspberry Almond Crumble Bars
8	Tomato Basil Mozzarella Frittata	Broccoli and Chicken Quiche	Chicken and Broccoli Casserole	Lemon Poppy Seed Almond Cake
9	Cauliflower Hash Browns	Pesto Zoodles with Cherry Tomatoes	Spinach and Feta Stuffed Chicken Breast	Coconut and Lime Sorbet
10	Turkey and Veggie Breakfast Skillet	Shrimp and Vegetable Skewers	Chickpea and Vegetable Curry	Greek Yogurt and Honey Frozen Drops
11	Avocado and Egg Toast	Tomato Basil Chicken Wrap	Teriyaki Tofu Stir-Fry	Mixed Berry Sorbet
12	Apple Cinnamon Quinoa Porridge	Cucumber and Radish Salad with Feta	Spaghetti Squash with Tomato Basil Sauce	Cinnamon Roasted Almonds
13	Egg and Veggie Breakfast Burrito	Minestrone Soup with Whole Wheat Pasta	Pesto Chicken with Roasted Vegetables	Ricotta and Berry Parfait
14	Smoked Salmon and Cucumber Wrap	Grilled Chicken Salad with Vinaigrette	Turkey and Vegetable Skillet	Baked Apples with Cinnamon
15	Oat Bran Porridge with Cinnamon	Spinach and Feta Turkey Burger	Broiled Lemon Garlic Tilapia	Strawberry and Mint Infused Water
16	Quinoa Breakfast Bowl	Turkey Lettuce Wraps	Greek Quinoa Salad	Almond Flour Blueberry Muffins
17	Mexican Breakfast Casserole	Quinoa and Black Bean Stuffed Peppers	Cauliflower and Lentil Curry	Coconut and Lime Sorbet
18	Peanut Butter Banana Smoothie	Mediterranean Chickpea Salad	Grilled Salmon with Dill Sauce	Chocolate Avocado Mousse

19	Zucchini and Cheese Egg Bake	Salmon and Asparagus Foil Packets	Zucchini Noodles with Pesto and Cherry Tomatoes	Pecan and Date Energy Squares
20	Avocado and Egg Toast	Spinach and Feta Turkey Burger	Chicken and Broccoli Casserole	Baked Pears with Cinnamon and Walnuts
21	Turkey and Veggie Breakfast Skillet	Cauliflower Rice Stir-Fry with Tofu	Lemon Garlic Shrimp Skewers	Vanilla Bean Panna Cotta
22	Quinoa Breakfast Bowl	Turkey and Avocado Wrap	Teriyaki Tofu Stir-Fry	Raspberry Almond Crumble Bars
23	Overnight Oats with Nuts and Berries	Grilled Veggie and Hummus Wrap	Greek Quinoa Salad	Pistachio and Cranberry Biscotti
24	Almond Flour Pancakes	Broccoli and Chicken Quiche	Chickpea and Vegetable Curry	Coconut and Lime Sorbet
25	Banana Walnut Muffins	Pesto Zoodles with Cherry Tomatoes	Spinach and Feta Stuffed Chicken Breast	Dark Chocolate-Dipped Strawberries
26	Berry and Spinach Smoothie Bowl	Tomato Basil Chicken Wrap	Spaghetti Squash with Tomato Basil Sauce	Greek Yogurt and Honey Frozen Drops
27	Tomato Basil Mozzarella Frittata	Minestrone Soup with Whole Wheat Pasta	Quinoa-Stuffed Bell Peppers	Baked Apples with Cinnamon
28	Cauliflower Hash Browns	Grilled Chicken Salad with Vinaigrette	Grilled Salmon with Dill Sauce	Lemon Poppy Seed Almond Cake
29	Turkey and Veggie Breakfast Skillet	Tuna Salad Lettuce Wraps	Teriyaki Tofu Stir-Fry	Almond and Coconut Energy Balls
30	Avocado and Egg Toast	Caprese Salad with Balsamic Glaze	Chickpea and Vegetable Curry	Mixed Berry Sorbet

Conversion Table

Volume Equivalents (Liquid)

US Standard	US Standard (oz.)	Metric (approximate)
2 tbsps	1 fl. oz.	30 milliliter
¼ cup	2 fl. oz.	60 milliliter
½ cup	4 fl. oz.	120 milliliter
1 cup	8 fl. oz.	240 milliliter
1½ cups	12 fl. oz.	355 milliliter
2 cups or 1 pint	16 fl. oz.	475 milliliter
4 cups or 1 quart	32 fl. oz.	1 Liter
1 gallon	128 fl. oz.	4 Liter

Volume Equivalents (Dry)

US Standard	Metric (approximate)
⅛ tsp	0.5 milliliter
¼ tsp	1 milliliter
½ tsp	2 milliliter
¾ tsp	4 milliliter
1 tsp	5 milliliter
1 tbsp	15 milliliter
¼ cup	59 milliliter
⅓ cup	79 milliliter
½ cup	118 milliliter
⅔ cup	156 milliliter
¾ cup	177 milliliter
1 cup	235 milliliter
2 cups or 1 pint	475 milliliter
3 cups	700 milliliter
4 cups or 1 quart	1 Liter

Oven Temperatures

Fahrenheit (F)	Celsius (C) (approximate)
250 deg.F	120 deg.C
300 deg.F	150 deg.C
325 deg.F	165 deg.C
350 deg.F	180 deg.C
375 deg.F	190 deg.C
400 deg.F	200 deg.C
425 deg.F	220 deg.C
450 deg.F	230 deg.C

Weight Equivalents

US Standard	Metric (approximate)
1 tbsp	15 gm
½ oz.	15 gm
1 oz.	30 gm
2 oz.	60 gm
4 oz.	115 gm
8 oz.	225 gm
12 oz.	340 gm
16 oz. or 1 lb.	455 gm

Conclusion

In conclusion, Type 2 diabetes is a long-term health issue where the body has trouble using insulin, leading to high sugar levels in the blood. It can cause serious problems, so it's important to handle it carefully. Your lifestyle, like what you eat and how much you exercise, plays a big part in managing and even turning around Type 2 diabetes.

This book is a helpful guide for people who want to take charge of their health and deal with Type 2 diabetes effectively. By trying out the recipes in the book, you can relish tasty food that's good for you. The recipes focus on wholesome, nutrient-packed foods that help keep your blood sugar stable and improve your overall well-being.

The recipes featured in this book are not only flavorful but also designed to align with dietary principles that support diabetes management. From nutrient-rich vegetables to lean proteins and wholesome grains, each recipe aims to strike a balance between taste and health. Moreover, the inclusion of a variety of components ensures a diverse and satisfying culinary experience, making it easier for individuals to adhere to a diabetes-friendly diet.

By embracing the recipes and nutritional guidance offered in this book, individuals can proactively make positive changes to their diet and lifestyle. Consistency in adopting these practices can contribute to better blood sugar control, weight management, and overall health improvement. Remember, it's not just about managing diabetes; it's about thriving and enjoying a fulfilling life.

Embark on this culinary adventure within the pages of this book, discovering the joy of nourishing your body while managing Type 2 diabetes effectively. Your journey to a healthier, more vibrant life starts with the first delicious bite – savor the flavors, embrace the nutrition, and empower yourself to take charge of your well-being. Here's to a year of renewed health and countless more to come!

Printed in Great Britain
by Amazon

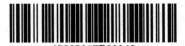

45663017R00048